The Origins of Bioethics

RHETORIC AND PUBLIC AFFAIRS SERIES

THE ORIGINS OF BIOETHICS

REMEMBERING WHEN MEDICINE WENT WRONG

John A. Lynch

MICHIGAN STATE UNIVERSITY PRESS | *East Lansing*

Michigan State University Press
East Lansing, Michigan 48823–5245

Printed and bound in the United States of America.

28 27 26 25 24 23 22 21 20 19   1 2 3 4 5 6 7 8 9 10

Library of Congress Cataloging-in-Publication Data is available
Names: Lynch, John (John Alexander), 1976– author.
Title: The origins of bioethics : remembering when medicine went wrong / John A. Lynch.
Description: East Lansing : Michigan State University Press, [2019]
| Series: Rhetoric and public affairs series | Includes bibliographical references and index.
Identifiers: LCCN 2018059493| ISBN 9781611863413 (pbk. : alk. paper)
| ISBN 9781609176174 (PDF) | ISBN 9781628953800 (ePub) | ISBN 9781628963816 (Kindle)
Subjects: LCSH: Human experimentation in medicine—Moral and ethical aspects—
United States—History. | Human experimentation in medicine—United States—Case studies.
| Medical ethics—United States—History. | Collective memory—Moral and ethical aspects—
United States—History. | Memorialization—Moral and ethical aspects—United States—History.
Classification: LCC R853.H8 L96 2019 | DDC 174.2/8—dc23
LC record available at https://lccn.loc.gov/2018059493

Book design by Charlie Sharp, Sharp Designs, East Lansing, MI
Cover design by Erin Kirk New
Cover photo from the administrative files of the Tuskegee Syphilis Study (ca. 1932–1972).
Courtesy of the National Archives at Atlanta.

Michigan State University Press is a member of the Green Press Initiative and is
committed to developing and encouraging ecologically responsible publishing
practices. For more information about the Green Press Initiative and the use
of recycled paper in book publishing, please visit *www.greenpressinitiative.org*.

Visit Michigan State University Press at *www.msupress.org*

Contents

———⋅◆⋅———

Acknowledgments

————•◆•————

As with my last book, this one is a product of serendipity and the encouragement of others, as much as any inspiration of my own. I had proposed a project for my first sabbatical, but then found myself bored by my own idea. After wracking my brain, I thought there might be something to say about the history and memory of the bioethics that I had been teaching at the University of Cincinnati's College of Medicine for the previous five years. I had doubts about the idea, until it received enthusiastic support from Jenell Johnson and Nathan Stormer. Their interest, encouragement, and continued conversation with me since then has sustained me and helped make this project what it is. Jenell and Lisa Corrigan both generously reviewed drafts of chapters in this project. Additionally, Leah Ceccarelli and Jeff Bennett have kindly listened to me talk about the challenges I faced working through this project, and as always, Celeste Condit has been a nurturing presence in my life and career. I can only hope to reflect, however dimly, her intellectual virtuosity and her generosity in mentorship.

I have also benefited from the opportunity to talk about this project with countless others. I had the opportunity to develop parts of this project at the Discourses of Health and Medicine Symposium at Cincinnati, Ohio, in 2015, and the feedback from my paper workshopping group—Teresa Thompson, Susan Wells, Barbara Heifferon, and Lisa Meloncon—improved the work I did on Willowbrook's bioethical memory. I had the opportunity to further hone the public memory components of this project at the Rhetoric Society of America's seminar "The Rhetorical Spaces of Memory" at Bloomington, Indiana, in 2017. The guidance of the seminar leaders, Carole Blair and Greg Dickinson, was invaluable, and I valued the feedback I received at the seminar and from a project workshop group that included Harry Archer, Meredith Johnson, Nathan Johnson, Amy Lueck, and Candace Rai.

During my visits to the sites of memory examined here, I had gracious guides who made sure I did not miss anything of interest. I want to thank Jontyle Robinson and Stephen Sodeke from Tuskegee University and James Kaser from the College of Staten Island for conversation about the studies at Tuskegee and the Willowbrook School, respectively. I also want to thank Marty Medhurst and the two manuscript reviewers for their feedback and editorial guidance.

In addition to intellectual support, I need to acknowledge the financial support that has helped me complete this project. I want to thank Steve Depoe and the Department of Communication for the sabbatical that allowed me to complete the majority of the fieldwork for this project. I also need to thank the University of Cincinnati's Third Century Faculty Research Fellowship for release time in 2016 to complete an early draft of the book manuscript.

Writing about the events that led to bioethics is depressing, highlighting as it does how those with the noblest of intentions can produce the most horrific of outcomes. I have been sustained during this project by my families of blood and of choice. My aunt Claire Pancero has always encouraged my curiosity since I was a small child. I appreciate her sharing memories of David Jungnickel, one of the victims of the Cincinnati TBI study who lived next door to my maternal grandmother. My father, John A Lynch Jr., who passed away while this book was in production; my mother Karen Lynch; my sister Jill Lynch Atwood and her daughters Brynn, Katelyn, and Kylee; and my brother Andrew Lynch and his partner Russ Wintgens have all been wonderful and supportive. I must also thank my closest friends Jeremy and Lisa Boerger, who so graciously made my partner and I part of their family and uncles to their children Stephen, Roger, and Ilsa.

Finally, I want to thank my partner, John Baughcum, for continuing to put up with my foibles: You make my world brighter for being in it.

Introduction

————•◆•————

Whenn I—or you, or anyone—visit the doctor's office, I face a pile of forms to fill out and sign. Among those forms, there is at least one asking me to confirm that I consent to the examination and the treatments that will follow. Similarly, from 2008 to 2015, when I worked as a research ethics specialist, I would walk by a notice board asking people to participate in research. Those volunteers, along the way to joining a study, would be informed—in sometimes mind-numbing detail—about the study and asked to sign a document affirming their informed consent to participate.

It was not always this way. Since the time of Hippocrates, doctors have experimented and tinkered with the treatments they provided, based on their observations and experience.[1] In the twentieth century, as medicine become less an art and more a science, these brief experiments became increasingly bureaucratized and systematic, until they reached what is today considered the acme of medical research, the double-blind clinical trial.[2] The increase in organization did not alter radically the treatment of the subject or patient. They still had to depend on the goodwill of the doctor and his adherence (and it was almost always a "him") to the Hippocratic Oath to decide whether they would be in a study, what care they would receive, etc. Physicians even felt they had the *right* to experiment on patients, especially the indigent ones in public hospitals.[3]

Yet, doctors also realized that they needed to receive the permission of patients to use them for research.[4] This intensified in the middle of the twentieth century. The Nuremberg trials of Nazi doctors who had performed horrific experiments in the concentration camps led to the creation of the Nuremberg Code, a series of ten precepts to guide medical research. Physicians and researchers across the globe recognized the need for more protection of patients, which led to the World Medical Association's Declaration of Helsinki, published in 1964. The physician Henry Beecher published an article in the *New England Journal of Medicine* that identified more than twenty studies, published in that journal, that violated developing standards for consent as well as the best medical interests of the research subjects.[5] Yet, adherence to any standard for informed consent or consideration of beneficence was voluntary, and physicians resisted attempts to regulate clinical care and research. It was not until the early 1970s that the resistance faltered in the face of persistent legislative efforts to mandate informed consent. The impetus for this push was a series of controversies about medical research that shocked the nation. Some of these events have been memorialized both by medical professionals—clinicians, researchers, bioethicists, etc.—and by the general public, patient advocates, and others.

These events are moments where "medicine went wrong." What we remember out of the history of medical research and *how* we remember it is consequential for bioethics, for medical science, and for the general public. *The Origins of Bioethics: Remembering When Medicine Went Wrong* will examine the bioethical and public recall of these events. To accomplish this, I will focus on those events where memorials have been built and made accessible to the public. The case studies that make up the book—the Tuskegee Syphilis Study, the Willowbrook Hepatitis Study, and the Cincinnati Whole Body Radiation Study—highlight the dynamics behind how these events have been remembered and forgotten.

What's in a Name?

What does it mean to say these are cases where "medicine went wrong"? Why *this* name? It is not a common one in bioethical writing and teaching, where the term "research misconduct" is employed, but this bureaucratic language is relatively bloodless and fails to capture the visceral reaction and the outrage that arose when the public learned about these studies. "Research misconduct" also is used to discuss actions like improperly completing informed consent forms, not revealing financial conflicts of interest, and plagiarism. While these behaviors are problematic, they pale in comparison to the events that happened in Macon County, Alabama; at the Willowbrook State School on Staten Island; and at the radioisotope lab at Cincinnati General Hospital. Another possible term is "research crime." It was first used to describe the medical experiments conducted by the Nazis in the concentration camps, and it was repurposed by Stephen B. Thomas and Sandra Crouse Quinn to describe the Public Health Service's syphilis study in Tuskegee.[6] While the term likely reflects contemporary public attitudes, it is factually and critically problematic. First, the term fails to recognize that many in the medical community saw no ethical failing in the research at Willowbrook and Cincinnati (among other examples). They often rallied around the researchers at the time and still do to this day. Some even defend the U.S. Public Health Service's Tuskegee Syphilis Study.[7] Past and present resistance to the language of "research crime" is not solely the bailiwick of extremists. Those resisting are part of the medical and public mainstream. Public memory is, as Kendall Phillips tells us, about both blame *and* vindication.[8] If I called these events "research crimes" and equated them with Nazi medical experiments, I would render these debates about blame, regret, shame, and vindication opaque.

Instead of these options, I have turned to the language of "medicine gone wrong." I believe it helps us avoid the absolute judgment that comes with comparing any post-WWII event with the Nazis, while also sidestepping the lack of judgment and public feeling that comes with the language of "research misconduct." The phrase positively addresses the history and memory of these events. First, it recognizes that research we now condemn developed out of the "normal" modes of science—à la Thomas Kuhn, the workaday methodological, epistemological, *and ethical* presumptions for research—in a given time.[9] These normal modes of science allowed medical researchers to look past the ethical problems in their research because they were doing research that looked very much like the work being done by peers and contemporaries.

Second, while recognizing the role that "normal" medical science played in allowing these events to happen, it also keeps open the conceptual space for recognizing that not all medical researchers were blind to the ethical implications of normal medical research. They could recognize something troubling about the research being conducted. The sense of something "going wrong" mirrors what existentialists following Martin Heidegger call the *unheimlich* or the uncanny, which will be discussed further in chapter 1.[10] Medical researchers would experience this sense of the uncanny when they began to doubt the normal practices of science and began to feel that something was not right in how patients and research subjects were being treated. Some researchers, like Henry Beecher, clearly recognized the shortcomings of medical and research ethics and called for other researchers to acknowledge the shortcomings of the normal modes of medical research in the mid-twentieth century. Other researchers might have had a similar experience, since this same time period saw researchers begin grappling with issues of informed consent and research ethics, even as ethically troubling research continued.[11] Yet for many, this sense of the uncanny never reached the level of ethical contemplation. Instead, the researchers would claim that an ignorant and easily roused public misunderstood medical science. In this way, the sense of the uncanny was resolved by purifying the physician of doubts, which were displaced onto others whose concerns could be dismissed.

The language of "medicine gone wrong" then captures this historical and contemporary wrangle of guilt, blame, and absolution focused on biomedical research.

Medical Science in the Mid-twentieth Century

In a number of cases like Tuskegee, Willowbrook, and Cincinnati, medical researchers grounded in the normal modes of science failed to see that the work they were doing harmed the dignity, rights, and bodies of diverse others. Calling this "normal science" is accurate but insufficient. It still leaves unanswered the question of *what* was normal then, which in turn might help explain *why* researchers and their science went wrong. Medical research in the first two-thirds of the twentieth century can be delimited by two factors.

The first factor is the professionalization of medicine that started in the mid-nineteenth century.[12] At that time, a multitude of medical schools existed in the United States, each offering a different school or perspective on the practice of medicine. The bar to entering the medical profession was quite low: there were no requirements for prior education, and individuals who had not yet completed high school could enroll in some medical schools. This situation began to change when some German-trained American doctors began advocating for the German model of medical education. The German model was based on an education in biological sciences, including substantial laboratory work, followed by practical clinical experience. This model, taken up by the American Medical Association, was promoted nationwide. It led to increasing standards for admission to medical schools and the development of state licensure and certification of doctors. It culminated in the 1910 Flexner Report, which accelerated the trend toward higher admission standards to medical schools and increased certification nationwide. In addition to eliminating almost all of the schools dedicated to what we today call "complementary and alternative medicine," it also led to the closure of five of the seven medical schools dedicated to training African American doctors.

Professionalization resulted in autonomy for medical doctors and researchers. According to James H. Jones, "by the 1930s, medicine had emerged as an autonomous, self-regulating profession whose members were in firm control of the terms, conditions, content, and goals of their work."[13] This held doubly true for medical researchers, and Jones argues that "there was no system of normative ethics on human experimentation during the 1930s."[14] Despite this formal lack, Susan Lederer notes, "Researchers observed limits in their experiments with human subjects. Although lacking enforcement policies . . . ethical guidelines influenced the conduct of research."[15] Those guidelines that did exist are epitomized in the Hippocratic Oath. According to Lisa Keränen, the rise of the Hippocratic Oath as the ubiquitous expression of medical ethics coincides with medicine's professionalization in the nineteenth century.[16] The Oath emphasized values of beneficence and non-maleficence (i.e., to help others and to do no harm) but lacked any concrete expression of what benevolence or non-maleficence meant in practice. It maintained "a paternalistic vision of medicine" where values of patient autonomy and informed consent were absent.[17] In other words, the abstract qualities of the Hippocratic Oath made it the perfect ethical expression for a system where medical researchers operated autonomously. Individual doctors determined what the most beneficial and least harmful course was for patients, with no input from the patients themselves.

While physician and researcher autonomy in charting the course of research and judging its ethical value were important, physicians and researchers were also influenced by larger cultural and social trends. According to Jordan Goodman, Anthony McElligott, and Lara Marks, "the concept of *usefulness* is the point of contact between human experimentation, knowledge, and the state. . . . The modern state increasingly used its prerogative to lay claim to the individual body for its own needs, whether social, economic, or military."[18] Usefulness is a specific articulation of biopower that emphasized the direct employment of bodies toward the ends of the state: Individuals had to be usable and were valued to the degree that they contributed economically, militarily, or reproductively to the state. Those who could not work and those who could not reproduce had to be rendered *usable*. Goodman and colleagues make this logic explicit: "For much of the twentieth century, the use of the experiment as a means of changing useless to useful revolved around using prisoners, orphans and hospital inmates as material."[19] Bodies had to be usable. Those who could not work because of increasing illness or developmental disability—or those whose work was not valued because of racism—were made usable through medical research.

Attempts to render bodies usable dovetailed with medical professionalization. Medical researchers were recruited into the state's mission of usability, and in exercising their prerogatives as medical researchers, they determined who would be made usable and how that would occur. As Susan Lederer notes, medical doctors and researchers had ethical impulses and discussed ethical issues, but they never progressed from private ethical talk to developing an ethical framework to guide their work. Changes in this attitude only began appearing in the late 1960s, and that change took more than a decade to bear fruit.[20] Medical professionalization and the state's demands for the usability of its citizens' bodies created the milieu in which medical research went astray and harmed those it was supposed to help. The history of medical research is unfortunately replete with these ethical failings, which have been well documented by scholars in bioethics and history. Some of these many episodes were used explicitly to justify the creation of research regulations in the United States. Bioethics fashions a creation story around three major "horror stories" of American research: the Tuskegee Study of Untreated Syphilis; the Willowbrook Hepatitis Study; and the Jewish Chronic Disease Hospital Cancer Study. These three studies are framed as the impetus behind the creation of bioethics and research regulation. While other stories have risen to prominence in the past decade—the treatment of Henrietta Lacks and syphilis experiments in Guatemala being the most prominent—they have yet to attain the canonical status of these three.

When we examine memories of these events, though, they are not treated equally. The study in Tuskegee has two museums dedicated to it. Monuments to the Willowbrook State School and its closure exist, but the Willowbrook Hepatitis Study is rarely remembered in those spaces (although a short film exists that dramatizes the events of the study), and the Jewish Chronic Disease Hospital study is not publicly memorialized at all. In addition to these three major events, there are also research studies that are conspicuous in their absence from bioethical memory. One of these is the Cincinnati Whole Body Radiation Study (WBS). Senator Edward Kennedy (D-MA) took up the study in his attempt to place requirements for informed consent on biomedical research, but his quest was soon aborted and forgotten. Yet, there *is* a public memorial to the Cincinnati WBS, but ironically, it is a memorial that works to suppress public recollection of the study.

This book then will look at the processes of remembering and forgetting that circulate around three bioethical cases that have been memorialized in public: Tuskegee, Willowbrook, and Cincinnati. Part 1 provides the theory and historical context that frames the case studies. Chapter 1 begins with an examination of public memory scholarship to identify key qualities of the research that are complicated, altered, or amplified when we consider how bioethics and public memory intersect. Specifically, it identifies the contours of *bioethical* memory: the mnestic capacity of discourses and places to bear witness and assume responsibility for the failure of medical science to uphold its ethical commitments. Yet, that call to bear witness struggles with the desires of institutions to protect their reputation and image, leading states and universities to create moments of *minimal remembrance,* which involves thinning out the act of witnessing, downplaying the contents of memory to save an institution's reputation. Next, it situates the cases to be studied against the larger ethical and policy changes around research and research ethics in the middle of the twentieth century. Then, in part 2, the book examines three cases of bioethical memory and their instantiation in public space. Each case represents a point on an arc of attention, moving from the well-remembered and memorialized case of Tuskegee to the more-or-less forgotten case of the Cincinnati Whole Body Radiation Study.

The study at Tuskegee (popularly known as the "Tuskegee Syphilis Study") is the heart of the third chapter. It is prominently remembered in bioethics and in public. Bioethicists invoke its name when they want to raise a warning flag about a study, and for the public, its draw is so powerful that journalists describe almost all newly discovered cases of medical research abuse or medical racism as "just like Tuskegee."[21] The study is memorialized at two museums located in Tuskegee, Alabama. They offer competing public memories of the study: the Tuskegee History Center positions the study as central to understanding the region's past and as a key to understanding the civil rights activism that occurred in the region, while the Tuskegee University's Legacy Museum elides the details of the study to offer an extended meditation on the intertwined legacy of racism that marks the region and the legacy of the university's anti-racist activism.

Chapter 4 considers the Willowbrook Hepatitis Study, which occurred at the Willowbrook State School in Staten Island, New York. Developmentally disabled children were infected with hepatitis through the use of hepatitis-infected feces mixed into milk so that doctors could study the progression of the disease. The medical community rallied around the study's lead investigator, Saul Krugman. While this helped minimize memorialization of the study, the entire situation is overwhelmed by public memory of Willowbrook itself, an overcrowded, filthy place where the developmentally disabled were warehoused. Exposés of conditions at the school foster overwhelming feelings of horror and disgust at the conditions there, and those public feelings overwhelm some of the details of events at the school, like Krugman's study. Such horror also requires deft management by those who would memorialize the school so that this public feeling can be managed and channeled. State officials offer a minimal remembrance of the school: They aggrandize themselves for closing the school that they had let sink into squalor. Vernacular remembrance uses that public feeling of disgust and horror to reframe the (able-bodied) public's relationship to the developmentally disabled, but does so in ways that conform to problematic frames for representing disability. Against this backdrop, the chapter then examines the one extant instance of public memory focused on the Willowbrook Hepatitis Study, the short film *Willowbrook,* and how it sidesteps details about the study and the school in order to facilitate a sense of the unheimlich and encourage bioethical contemplation of the study.

Finally, the last chapter will study the Cincinnati Whole Body Radiation Study. This study is notable for the lack of memory and memory artifacts surrounding it. There have been repeated attempts to suppress details of the study—in other words, to forget it. While information about it is publicly available, the Cincinnati Whole Body Radiation Study lacks the material and symbolic support necessary to make it "bioethical memory." The undermining of that support occurred in two episodes. At one point in the early 1970s, the study was publicly revealed and compared to other instances where medicine had gone wrong, but it rapidly disappeared from public circulation. That meaningful forgetting allowed all parties in the controversy to gain something: requirements for informed consent in DOD research for congressional investigators and a secured reputation for the university and the researchers. The study again came to public attention in the 1990s. That public awareness led to a lawsuit by the families of the study's victims, and part of the university's settlement of that suit involved the creation of a memorial to individuals in the study. Yet that memorial is crafted and placed in such a way as to again undermine memory and foster forgetting.

In the conclusion, I summarize the findings of the study and consider the arc of memory and forgetting that characterizes the different ways in which episodes of medicine going wrong are remembered. I consider how these different memorial strategies reflect the various attempts at managing the identities and the public feelings of various audiences and how those strategies can inform both bioethical and rhetorical scholarship.

PART 1

Theory and History
of Bioethical Memory

CHAPTER 1

Bioethical Memory
and Minimal Remembrance

———•◆•———

I n the first two-thirds of the twentieth century, medical researchers
were professionalized to believe that their individual judgments
were sufficient to determine the most beneficial, least harmful course
for those in their clinical care and in their medical research. In offering
medical care and conducting medical research, they were guided by
demands that all bodies should be *useful* for the polity, even the bodies
of the ill and the developmentally disabled. Views about medical ethics
and usability changed, which led medical ethicists and the general public to decry some of the research being conducted in the United States.
Historically, some of those events became the impetus for changing how
medical research occurred in the United States and across the globe.
Those events are now recalled in numerous settings. Yet a tension exists between the demand to remember and equally salient demands on
the state and many institutions to preserve their reputation and image,
which would be harmed by the recollections of medical histories. Here I

draw from literature in rhetoric, public memory, and bioethics to outline the concepts of bioethical memory and minimal remembrance.

Bioethical Memory

The concept of bioethical memory builds on existing work on public memory in rhetorical studies. Public memory, as Carol Blair, Greg Dickinson, and Brian Ott argue, is "an activity of collectivity rather than (or in addition to) individuated, cognitive work . . . [that is] activated by present concerns, issues, or anxieties."[1] Thomas Dunn argues, "Within the frame of public memory, the past operates not as historical *fact* but as historical *interpretation* for the purposes of making public argument. Through framing the past, we serve a present need."[2] These definitions emphasize the mnestic (or memory-bearing) capacity of all symbolic- and material-rhetorical practices.[3] This mnestic capacity of all rhetoric is reflected in the range of artifacts that have been identified as examples of public memory, including books, speeches, photographs, television, and movies; but the most prominent memory artifacts are often memorials and museums.[4] These projects highlight how memories are partial and often contested.[5] Any single memory is limited and only able to encapsulate part of the past, typically those parts the display of which would benefit the people crafting the memory or reflect the dominant values of the broader culture.

While it draws on these general qualities of public memory, bioethical public memory mobilizes the mnestic capacities of rhetoric in order to bear witness to the past. According to Barbie Zelizer, bearing witness means to "assume responsibility for the events of our times. . . . Bearing witness constitutes a specific form of collective remembering that interprets an event as significant and deserving of critical attention."[6] The critical attention that comes from witnessing requires individuals "to understand and verbalize the lessons of injustice and tragedy" and also to act on those lessons.[7] For Zelizer, bearing witness combines historical truth-telling and interpretation: We make an argument in the present for why collective witnessing of the past is crucial to our values and identities in the present day. This leaves open space for contestation and disagreement, but this does not undermine witnessing. As Zelizer argues, "bearing witness implies that there is no best way of depicting or thinking about atrocities, but that the very fact of paying heed collectively is crucial."[8] Bioethicist and narrative medicine scholar Arthur Frank argues that bioethics, especially a bioethics defined by a narrative focus, has a duty to "witness suffering."[9] To further develop the concept of bioethical memory, we must consider how the act of bearing witness modifies how identity and emotion, as well as materiality and symbolicity, operate in public memory.

IDENTITY AND EMOTION

Two key qualities of public memory are their role in creating shared identities and the mobilization of public feeling to secure adherence to the identities provided. Blair and colleagues emphasize identity as a key outcome of public memory. For them, public memory narrates "a common identity, a construction that forwards an at least momentarily definitive articulation of the group."[10] The partiality of memory and the resultant competition make public memory a nexus "where a host of rhetors and audiences are involved in the performative process of individual and collective identity."[11] Public memory "is always there to be *invoked*," to reassure us about our national, regional, or professional identities.[12] It also plays a key role in our senses of race and gender, sharpening the identities offered by those categories as well.[13] It also configures the relationship that collective identity has to the past, especially the responsibility or culpability those constituted by that identity must assume.[14]

Memory offers us narratives that shape collective identities, but those narratives qua narrative do not guarantee that collectives will adhere to the identities offered in those narratives. "It is not enough, for example to say that those vehicles of memory are narratives or rituals or relics," Blair and colleagues note, "because some narratives, rituals, and relics secure more collective attachment than others."[15] One of the most important qualities of public memory that secures collective support for narratives is the animation of that memory by public feeling. In using the language of "public feeling," I am following Debra Hawhee and Jenell Johnson in preferring the term over the more common conceptual dichotomy of affect and emotion.[16]

Following Brian Massumi, rhetorical scholars often argue for the difference between affect, framed as nonconscious intensities, and emotion, which is the articulation of that affective intensity within systems of meaning.[17] Hawhee argues that discussions of affect and emotion in rhetorical scholarship tend to stop at "rehearsing the accepted division between emotion and affect as known and inchoate respectively."[18] Johnson argues that "feeling" better addresses "the complex relationship between bodily intensity, the perception of that intensity, and its translation into language," especially in historical analyses where "we only have access to the feelings of the past through their recorded expression—the same textual traces that tell us a public was here."[19] The uncertainty and ephemerality implied by the term "feeling" is especially appropriate for attempts to assess memories of events that evoked the morass of feelings that many associated with medical research tried (often successfully) to repress.

Specifically, feeling animates the narratives of public memory, facilitating adherence to the details of the events described and the identities or subject positions offered to the audiences of the narrative. Following Sarah Ahmed, we can ask, "what sticks?" in the narratives of events where medicine went wrong.[20] Blair and colleagues identify two levels at which public feeling operates: They "suggest that what Aristotle called *philia,* and what we might label affiliation, is, by definition, the principal affective modality of public memory."[21] This collective sense of belonging, as well as the individual's own degree of attachment to that collective, is facilitated by many things, including other public feelings "like pride, contempt, anxiety, anger, horror, shame, guilt, confidence, gratitude, or compassion . . . [that] contribute to the production and maintenance of affiliation in more or less direct ways, in various configurations, and with various investments."[22]

Yet, public feelings, especially *philia,* need further elaboration. Blair and colleagues ground their perspective on philia in Aristotle's *Rhetoric,* but as Eugene Garver notes, Aristotle's definition of the passions in the *Rhetoric,* among which he includes philia, differs somewhat from his discussion elsewhere.[23] Philia is also a topic in the *Politics* and the *Nichomachean Ethics.* In the *Rhetoric,* philia is a public feeling used in appealing to one's audience (1380b34–1381a10), but elsewhere Aristotle offers a more expansive definition of it as "some sort of excellence or virtue, or involves virtue, and it is, moreover, most indispensable for life" (1155a4–5).[24] As Eleni Leontsini argues, philia (or civic friendship) "is important because it contributes to the unity of both the state and community by transmitting feelings of intimacy and solidarity."[25] These feelings of intimacy and solidarity are a necessary component of ethics and justice, a point first made by Aristotle and reinforced by contemporary commentary on his work.[26]

An additional quality of philia not raised by the *Rhetoric* is the role of *homonoia,* translated as concord or consensus, which is the condition "when the citizens have the same judgment about their common interest, when they choose the same things, and when they execute what they have decided in common" (Aristotle, *Nichomachean Ethics,* 1167a25–29). Garver describes it as "more a matter of knowing *how* than knowing *that.*"[27] Concord is an essential component of philia: In order to have feelings of intimacy and solidarity, it is necessary to have some core around which that intimacy and solidarity develops. In other words, homonoia or concord is the Aristotelian way of emphasizing the identity that is at the heart of public memory. Further, the classical discussion of philia and homonoia underscores the fundamental unity of identity and emotion in public memory scholarship. People become invested in the identities offered by public memory because of the sense of philia or affiliation with that memory and its attendant identity. To have philia or affiliation is to already have an identification with a group and a set of ideals associated with them.

In bioethical memory, one assumes the identity of witness, joining a collective that agrees an event is deserving of critical attention. That affiliation with other witnesses to bioethical events is enabled in various ways by feelings ranging from pride to horror to shame to compassion. This philia is one among many affiliations or identities any individual witness will possess, and the character of one's bearing witness will be inflected by the other roles one inhabits, like doctor or patient. Medical doctors affiliate among themselves, creating a community that identifies broadly with the institution of medicine and defends it against attacks from outsiders. They invest in an identity framed by benevolent exercise of medical knowledge. Yet, this community of doctors—a collective sharing of an identity that sticks as a result of affiliation/philia made possible or facilitated by years of clinical training—exists in relationship to others. This is reflected synecdochically in the Hippocratic Oath, where the relationships of doctors to patients are articulated. This relationship is a key quality of the philia of many bioethical memories: We are called to bear witness to how this relationship sometimes goes astray, and to account for the psychic distress it causes patients and communities, as well as the medical doctors. This distress is reflected in other public feelings that can complicate philia. As Garver notes, "we judge the actions of others differently when colored by shame, benevolence, pity, or envy."[28] Three emotions are noteworthy for bioethical memory: disgust, anger, and the *unheimlich.*

Medical science involves bodies in various forms of distress—sickened, sometimes bedridden, occasionally filthy, and too frequently in pain. Many reactions are possible, but a common one would be disgust. As Sara Ahmed notes, disgust is often aroused by perceptions of filth or dirtiness and nakedness.[29] The articulation of disgust moves through three moments. First, one experiences an initial reaction of pulling away, that what initiated the response "threatens to stick to us."[30] Second, one makes that disgust apparent through facial and bodily comportment or a verbal declaration (e.g., "That's disgusting!"). Third, one distances oneself from the object or individuals to whom disgust adheres: Ahmed describes this third step as the move to declare, "'They are disgusting,' which translates into, 'We are disgusted by them.'"[31] This is one potential reaction to bodies, especially those bodies that have been neglected or abused by those who should otherwise care for them. Problematic medical research elicits expressions of horror and outrage, which are the translation of disgust into rhetorical distance from that research. This processing of disgust and horror thus facilitates philia: we witnesses are united in our disgust. Yet, the affective economy of disgust is problematic. In its move to distance the shared subject that feels disgust from the Other or object to which disgustingness gets attributed, "disgust might not allow one to get close enough to an object before one is compelled to pull away."[32] Disgust creates a collective identity that, in their rejection of the disgusting thing, might improve conditions for those harmed (e.g., "We must close down this disgusting institution!" or "We must stop this type of disgusting research!"). Yet, disgust simultaneously has the capacity to foreclose further engagement with the issue: Instead of being disgusted at the conditions in which people have been placed, we might reject the people, doubling the harms they experience.

Disgust can be a powerful motivator, and its capacity to affect those bearing witness is complemented by anger. Ahmed argues that anger can arise in response to witnessing pain, and I believe it can also occur in response to disgusting situations. Anger can be unproductive—"there are moments of anger where it is unclear what one is angry about"[33]—and can be used as a defense against legitimate (bio)ethical claims about injustice; but anger can also contribute to progressive missions of social justice. Ahmed draws on feminist and black feminist scholarship to outline anger's productive ethical capacity. According to Ahmed, "Crucially, anger is not simply defined in relationship to a past, but as opening up the future. . . . Being against something is also being for something, but something that has yet to be articulated or is not yet."[34] Here, anger is a response to past injustice that becomes the motivating force that both informs and drives those who feel it toward a better future. This type of anger that motivates witnesses to remedy past actions is a productive and ethical emotion.

Another key public feeling is the uncanny. According to Michael Hyde, the sense of the uncanny (the unheimlich) strips away our sense of familiarity with our world and our routines.[35] In the experience of the uncanny and the anxiety it produces, Hyde notes, "No psychological distance exists between our 'selves' and what this emotion reveals."[36] The immediacy of the uncanny calls into question our ability to navigate our lives; in other words, the know-how that helps constitute homonoia/concord becomes disturbed. Unlike disgust and anger, which create distance between the self and other, the uncanny does not allow the creation of psychological distance to separate us from the source of our anxiety and loss. Rather than action directed outward at conditions, people, or events we find problematic, the unheimlich directs the person's attention inward toward self-reflection. In this way, the unheimlich can be ethically transformative, as individuals assess their identities, affiliations, and actions and change them in response to that unheimlich-driven reflection. Clearly, this capacity would be valuable for bioethics: Encouraging clinicians and researchers to reflect on their actions, how they impact patients and research subjects, and then change those behaviors is a laudable goal for bioethics. Yet, the unheimlich, like anger and disgust, can have ethically problematic impacts. In his study of the suburbs, Greg Dickinson notes that suburban life is driven by a sense of unheimlich.[37] The uncanny produces nostalgia, which leads people to pursue "never-existing objects"—times, places, and modes of life that never existed outside of collective fantasy—through destructive consumerist practices.[38] Similarly, when faced with the unheimlich, medical practitioners and researchers might reject that experience. During their training, health-care providers, especially medical doctors, have been trained to practice "clinical detachment" or "detached concern," where they constrain their own emotional responses in order to provide competent medical care.[39] An individual might reject the uncanny as creating doubt and uncertainty, undermining the ability to provide competent care. Such a reaction is possible when the unheimlich balances those who experience it on the knife edge between ethical self-reflection described by Hyde and the nostalgia and melancholic search for an object that never was that Dickinson described.

Overall, philia encapsulates both the public feeling of solidarity and intimacy that develops around the identities—the homonoia or concord—in public and bioethical memory. Those identities are facilitated by a variety of emotions, including disgust, anger, and the unheimlich. The key identity of bioethical memory is that of witness, but while witnessing is key for the public as a whole, witnesses also still maintain other identities and roles. Some of those, like medical professionals, might find those identities strengthened, questioned, or diminished by what they witness. The act of witnessing also creates the grounds upon which calls for ethical, legal, and social change can be made. Witnesses not only critically attend to an event but work to safeguard people in the present and future against similar events.

MATERIAL AND SYMBOLIC SUPPORTS

Memories narrate an identity as witness and are animated by public feeling, which helps those identities "stick" for those who encounter them, but they also require a variety of material and symbolic supports. First, memory requires conditions of publicity. This means more than the information being generally accessible. As Rosa Eberly observes in her analysis of radio talk shows about the University of Texas tower shootings,

> While the radio makes discourse public, it does not make public discourse. That is, radio gives public access, but it does not necessarily lead to public discourse—to private people discoursing together in public about shared consequences, collective judgment, and conjoint action.[40]

Like public discourse, memories must become the focus of collective action and judgment to become public. Yet, publicity alone is not sufficient for making public memory. Public memory has a specific range of symbolic and material forms. Both Charles E. Scott and Barbie Zelizer argue that middle voice is vital to public memory. Voice, according to Zelizer, "is defined grammatically as that which shows the relationship between the subject and the word of action in a statement."[41] Scott emphasizes that middle-voice constructions are neither passive nor active, and they "are most appropriate when we speak of events of public memory with primary attention . . . to ways public memory appears and takes place."[42] Voice helps create the relationship between people and the contents of memory.

Among the many symbolic and material supports for memory, place might be one of the most important and unique. Edward S. Casey argues that public memory is enacted in places: "This is more than a matter of setting; it is a question of an active material *inducement* by the place—its power of drawing out the appropriate memories in that location."[43] Place acts as a vital rhetorical resource for public memory in several ways. First, place acts as the signifier for public memory. As Blair and colleagues argue, "The signifier—the place—is an object of attention and desire. It is an object of attention because of its status as a place, recognizable and set apart from undifferentiated space."[44] At its most basic, "the place tells us something was there."[45] The creation and designation of a place *as* a place of public memory also emphasizes that something important happened in or near that place: The various costs of construction, political wherewithal to designate a site as one of historic or cultural importance, etc., limits the creation of public memory spaces and amplifies any given place's importance.[46] Alongside their cost and rarity, places of public memory are unique in that they cannot be moved; individuals must travel to memorials, museums, and other memory spaces, necessitating "a particular set of performances on the part of people who would seek to be its audience."[47] Place qua place is important, as the nomination of a place as a site of public memory indicates that something happened worthy of our attention, which requires individuals to make specific arrangements to travel and engage with the place.

Place itself also has a role in constructing the temporal aspect of identities developed by public memory. First, the stability of a specific place might create a sense of its permanence and immutability, thus helping to foster a sense of community with the past: Visiting a stable, seemingly immutable space of historic significance can foster for visitors a sense of co-presence with those historical individuals and events.[48]

Memory places also create connections to others in the present: "What is palpably different about the rhetoric of memory places, though, is the recognizability of other visitors at the site. The visitor is not just imagining connections to people of the past, but experiencing connections to people in the present."[49] At its most basic, the recognition that others have been drawn to a site of memory creates the public feeling of philia or affiliation central to public memory, thus contributing to other narrative, symbolic, and material attempts to foster that feeling.

These qualities of place are undoubtedly true for many memorials and museums, but they are complicated for bioethical memory by its operation across the public and technical spheres. Bioethical memory existing in public spaces draws on the material and symbolic supports common to all public memory, but bioethical memory in the technical sphere of medicine and biomedical research is most frequently performed in a classroom setting. As Susan Reverby argues, bioethics training courses for medical researchers start with the "series of begats," a bioethics creation story of how events like Tuskegee and Willowbrook led to the Belmont Report, IRBs (institutional review boards), and the regulatory panoply of modern research oversight.[50] The stories offered create the past as the justification for bioethics and IRBs, and they shape the identity of medical researchers and bioethicists in the present. The stories position students as witnesses to the horrors of pre-bioethics research and then positions them as the individuals whose right action, in accordance with bioethical values and research regulation, safeguards against a return to problematic research. The bioethics classroom—whether physical or virtual—melds memory, identity, and education. In doing so, it is like the museums that are often the focus of rhetorical public memory studies, but the bioethics classroom does not partake of the power typical of memory spaces. It is not a unique signifier that demands unique plans to travel and to visit. It does not situate us in a place where historic events occurred. The classroom is a multiplicity: It is repeated across institutions with each class space being substantially identical, and with online bioethics and RCR (responsible conduct of research) courses, even the demands of the physical classroom space—one must make time to get to campus and enter the classroom, etc.—are eliminated. Timing is further altered by the timing and delivery of course lectures: It is shaped by the demands of the academic year and not influenced by anniversaries of the events remembered. The multiplicity of the classroom also connotes a degree of fragmentation and partiality: What is taught and remembered in those spaces, while broadly conforming to the narratives circulating in the technical sphere of medical research, is also influenced by the concerns of individual teachers and by the biases of available textbooks.

Because of the tensions existing between public memory places and bioethical memory places, a rhetorical study of memories of bio-ethical lapses must work across these places and the different material and symbolic entailments of both. Such a study can inform bioethics by considering how and in what conditions the events that led to bioethics and research regulation are remembered by the public, but such a study will also encourage rhetoricians to recognize that some memory places are transitory and the value assigned to them can differ markedly.

Minimal Remembrance

Bearing witness is hard. It challenges extant group identities and threatens reputations, especially the reputations of storied institutions. Who wants to be known as the group or institution that gave us Tuskegee or Willowbrook? Yet institutions that housed some of the questionable research of the twentieth century play a role in shaping public memory of events that can harm the reputation and image of these institutions. Thus, bearing witness can run counter to other institutional imperatives, creating a desire to minimize memory—to produce memory artifacts that nominally remember an event but foster forgetting. On one level, this conflict manifests as the difference between "official" and "vernacular" memories.[51] According to Thomas Dunn, "State or public authorities articulate official public memories to solidify national, cultural, and community identities by shaping collective imaginings," and "vernacular memories articulate contrasting narratives of the past that serve local needs to a greater extent than official memory."[52]

Yet, this situation is more than a mere difference between official and vernacular memories. Bioethical memory's call to bear witness and the institution's need for self-preservation, promotion, and image management are in tension. This leads to what I call *minimal remembrance:* the crafting of memories sufficient to address historical and ongoing outcry about an event, yet thin enough to minimize harm to the institution's reputation. Minimal remembrance has similarities to Barbie Zelizer's "remembering to forget," the practice where bearing witness becomes thin and "ruptures the connection between representation and responsibility."[53] Minimal remembrance operates like remembering to forget in that it similarly ruptures the connection between representation and responsibility by reducing the responsibility of the witness. Yet it differs in two key ways. First, minimal remembrance goes beyond the rupture of representation and responsibility by working to minimize the blame that adheres to institutions historically involved with problematic medical practice and research. Reducing the blame attributable to the institution often involves minimizing the problematic aspects of the research, and this in turn reduces the need of witnesses to observe and respond to injustice. Second, minimal remembrance focuses attention on how the various political and social forces operating in institutions and organizations manifest in the creation and articulation of bioethical memories, as well as other forms of public memory that emphasize bearing witness. This differs from remembering to forget where "the act of bearing witness is growing thin," regardless of the specific content or institutional context of memory.[54] Zelizer's remembering to forget indicts media and social practice, while minimal remembrance criticizes the institutions that house bioethical memory. Previous work on the types of public memory and history and work on forgetting help define the contours of minimal remembrance.

HISTORY AND TYPES OF MEMORY

Because minimal remembrance is shaped by institutional concerns about image and reputation, the collective memory and self-identity of the institution and related groups, alongside the history of those groups and the event being witnessed, are thrown into sharp relief.

Different groups and collectives that are not fully "public" have memories. This quality of memory is reflected in a tension between individualistic and collectivistic "strains" of memory scholarship.[55] Jeffrey Olick delineates those two "strains." Individualistic strains of memory scholarship emphasize that only individuals have memory, although "group memberships provide the materials for memory and prod the individual into recalling particular events and into forgetting others," and collectivist strains emphasize that "memories are generalized *imagos*" that "are as much the products of the symbols and narratives available publicly—and of the social means for storing and transmitting them—as they are the possessions of individuals."[56]

Following Edward Casey, we can resolve this tension by parsing out four distinct forms of memory. At a base level, there is the individual's memory of events and experiences. It is followed by *social memory,* the "memory held in common by those who are affiliated, either by kinship ties, by geographical proximity in neighborhoods . . . or by engagement in a common project. In other words, it is memory shared by those who are *already* related to each other."[57] These are memories developed by those existing in a relationship, like an institution, or those given similar training and occupational identities, like doctors, which reaffirm the history and quality of their group identity. Examples of social memory are the recollections of African American families in Tuskegee, Alabama, about a family member's experience as a subject of the syphilis study, or the recollection of faculty at the University of Cincinnati's College of Medicine about the radiation experiments conducted there in the 1960s. Another form is *collective memory,* "the circumstance in which different persons, not necessarily known to each other at all, nevertheless recall the same event—again, each in her own way."[58] The key quality is that collective memory is radically polysemous; it is a "plural memory that has no basis in overlapping historicities or shared places but is brought together only in and by a conjoint remembrance of a certain event."[59] An exemplar of collective memory is the "flashbulb memory" of events like Kennedy's assassination or 9/11, and a bioethical example would be individuals recalling first seeing the news stories revealing the existence of the Tuskegee Syphilis Study or the horrific conditions at the Willowbrook State School.

Individual, social, and collective memory all contribute to Casey's final form of memory—public memory. For Casey, public memory's "publicness" indicates it occurs "where discussion with others is possible . . . where one is exposed and vulnerable."[60] Public memory *engenders* common identities, in contrast to social memory that exists as a result of preexisting relationships. Public memory serves "as an encircling horizon" for public discourse, acting as a resource for discussion and for collective action, thus extending beyond collective memory by translating events publicly known into public discourse and then public memory.[61] Scholars of public memory in various disciplines turn to some or all of these forms and meanings of public memory. Blair and colleagues encourage rhetoricians to focus primarily on the designator "public": "We acknowledge the terminological variances make a difference, but we collapse under the sign of 'public memory' those studies taking the stance that beliefs about the past are shared among members of a group."[62]

Sidestepping issues of levels or types of memory works when focusing primarily on memorials in public spaces, but it is less viable when one is engaging with memory work that crosses group, institutional, and public contexts. For example, Susan Reverby notes that accounts of the Public Health Service Syphilis Study acted as a flashbulb memory for participants in the early debates on bioethics and research regulation that they used to justify their work: This *collective memory,* as Casey would label it, became a key driver for initial work on bioethics that would, in the decade after 1972, become incorporated into bioethics's broader public memory.[63] In contrast to this positive and productive example of memory work across different levels and contexts, minimal remembrance involves groups investing in social memory to trump the operation of memory at the level of the public, especially when it threatens the institution and its social memories.

Minimal remembrance also involves the relationship of memory and history. Here, scholars have offered a number of definitions of this relationship. Kerwin Lee Klein documents how memory first emerged as a "counter-concept" for history that promised to "rework history's boundaries."[64] Kendall Philips recounts how memory studies, beginning with Halbwachs and Nora, have tended to frame history "as a singular and authentic account of the past" that is "fixed" or "dead," and memory as "multiple, diverse, mutable, and competing accounts of past events," although poststructuralist critiques have undermined the sense of history as singular and monolithic.[65] A variety of scholars have grappled with this relationship and how to parse out different modes or forms of recollection, identifying some as "history" and others as "memory."[66] Despite variations in their assessments of the two, most scholars would agree with Marita Sturken's succinct assessment that memory and history are "entangled."[67]

This entanglement is amplified in bioethical memory and minimal remembrance in two ways. First, history and memory in bioethics have become so entangled that there is often no functional difference between the two. In her account of the study at Tuskegee, Reverby notes that "neither the public nor the health care communities thought about the Study as just history or just memory . . . memory brings the research community and the public together, as narratives of ethics and memories of oppression become interlocked."[68] In fact, in bioethics, "it is the very histories in their truncated forms that become the memories."[69] Second, the history of the events that gave birth to bioethics have altered social organization and group identities. As we will see in greater depth in subsequent chapters, these events transformed how research is conducted, changed the relationship between medical doctors and their patients and research subjects, redefined care for the developmentally disabled, and reinforced African American fears of medical racism. The changes to these relationships, the social organization of medicine, and the practices of medical research impact the identities of all these groups, and given memory's ties to identity and philia, these historical changes will filter into the public memories through which we bear witness to this past and to who we all, collectively, were in those times.

FORGETTING

If many institutions and groups had their druthers, they would prefer to go beyond minimal remembrance and consign memory of bioethical events to the trash heap of history. Minimal remembrance sits on a continuum between robust public memory and attempts to erase and forget the past. Many early studies of public memory emphasized that memory involved both remembering and forgetting. In 1989, David Thelan argued, "People depend on others to help them decide which experiences to forget and which to remember and what interpretation to place on experience."[70] Many studies emphasize that "forgetting is itself integral to public memory."[71] While many studies ground themselves in the pairing of remembering and forgetting, Blair and colleagues challenge the pairing's near-axiomatic status. They argue,

> We believe the remembering-forgetting dialectic has been employed as a stand-in or a simplistic restatement of the problem of representation in public memory studies. In other words, a failure to represent a particular content publicly is not a necessary, or even provisional, sign of forgetting. To suggest otherwise is to assume that all memory contents are represented publicly and/or that what is articulated publicly is an exhaustive map of memory contents. Either of those assumptions is theoretically indefensible and counterfactual.[72]

Yet, they note that doubts about the dialectic does not mean that memories are never forgotten or suppressed. Rather, the "conditions for remembering and forgetting vary," and the memory-forgetting dialectic "should be replaced by a more nuanced and evidence-grounded position that takes account of the status of particular memory articulations in relation to others, in particular contexts, with particular attention to the inventional operations that mediate that status."[73] Greg Dickinson, for example, turns to the language of "meaningful forgetting" as a way of identifying the more nuanced rhetorical contours of forgetting he identified in the suburban megachurch.[74]

Developing a more robust conception of forgetting in the context of public memory scholarship requires shifting how the operation of forgetting is conceived. This involves a move from an emphasis on *memories of publics* (the epistemic contents of public memory) to emphasize the *publicness of memory* (the processes by which any specific memory content becomes public memory).[75] To emphasize what is known or not known leads to a conceptual abyss: as Blair and colleagues note, "The domain of the 'forgotten' within this so-called dialectical pair is nearly infinite."[76] Forgetting is often framed as wiping the slate of memory clean or as amnesia. Both imply a degree of irreversibility to forgetting, but Brad Vivian cautions against these commonplace definitions of forgetting: "*Forgetting* and *amnesia,* regardless of ordinary usage in public affairs and popular psychology, are not obvious synonyms."[77] Vivian argues that "to forget, at its root, means to miss or lose one's hold. The word strongly connotes losing one's grasp of something, not the thing itself. . . . *Neglect* seems a more direct synonym for forgetting than *amnesia.*"[78]

Defining forgetting as something akin to neglect shifts discussions of forgetting away from the contents of public memory to the publicness of memory. Public memory and public forgetting do not invoke questions of knowledge (i.e., is something known?). Instead, they raise questions, as Sara Ahmed says of political emotion, of "what sticks?" The "stickiness" of public memory encourages us to focus our attention on the material, affective, and symbolic supports that make any given memory "public." Memories are made available *as memories* through the circulation of narratives in public discourse or the circulation of people through a space. Those encountering "public" memory contents are hailed in the middle voice in which public memory contents are cast. When those material and symbolic supports are undermined, the formal qualities of memories that make memories "sticky"—that enable their publicness and their recognition as memories—disappear. The memories no longer "stick" and are thus forgotten.

The drive to forget derives from issues of identity and public feeling. People do not encounter memories as blank slates. They come to them with extant identities and an associated repertoire of public feelings. The affective charge of a public memory might threaten existing identities and feelings, thus necessitating the drive to forget the memory. We can see the urge to forget in many legacy and history sites associated with the South, where certain accounts of racism threaten identities grounded in whiteness.[79] A similar dynamic is at play in bioethical memory. The identity of the biomedical profession has been, and for many still is, grounded in the ethical value of *primum non nocere,* which lies at the core of the Hippocratic Oath. Events like the syphilis study at Tuskegee and the conditions at Willowbrook directly challenge this core dictum of medical identity and ethics. Similarly, most groups and institutions do not want to be known for horrible events that have occurred in our past. The urge to minimize responsibility for these events is great—so great that groups and institutions might engage in acts of minimal remembrance, trying to downplay or neglect those memories. Some will go beyond the neglect of minimal remembrance and attempt to forget events from medical research's past. To engage in minimal remembrance means crafting a memory that reflects some aspects of the past while downplaying issues of blame. To engage in forgetting involves suppressing the circulation of memory narratives, positioning them in places where it is hard for bodies to traverse and encounter the memory, or undermining the memory contents by not framing them in the middle voice and subjunctive mood. Medicine as a profession and the institutions that house it have a vested interest in minimizing and potentially forgetting the sordid elements of its past.

Conclusion

Bioethical memory consists of bearing witness to past events in medicine and medical research and bearing the responsibility to bring critical attention to those events. Individuals are bound together as the collective of witnesses by philia, the concord or collective identity and knowing together that is at the heart of philia, and other emotions—like disgust, anger, and the uncanny—that help motivate those witnesses. Yet, the responsibility of witnesses is modulated by other identities and emotions. The responsibilities of medical professionals as witnesses differ from the responsibilities of the lay public. All have the responsibility to pay attention, but what that "attention" is and what actions are demanded of people change with their identities, roles, and relation to the institutions and practices that have led to problematic bioethical events.

This differing responsibility involves the obligation to maintain or create public memory, which is often the purview of the state and large institutions, but it also involves assuming blame for the historical events in question. Yet, no one wants to be known as the group that gave us Willowbrook or irradiated cancer patients or let African American men suffer from syphilis instead of curing them. These biomedical events, among others, can so threaten a group or institution's identity that the memory of that event must be minimized, if not outright forgotten.

Creating memory artifacts and places sufficient to address historical and current outrage over an event while maintaining an institution's reputation is shaped by three factors implicated in memory's types or levels and memory's relationship to history. First, the more notorious the event, the more detail will be required to avoid outrage at an apparent failure to bear witness in an appropriate fashion. This highlights the role of emotions that contribute to public outrage like disgust and anger in public and bioethical memory. Second, the impact of the event on social structure and group identities also influences the degree of minimization possible. The more an event changed social structures or identities of the public or key institutions and groups, the more that event must be remembered. This highlights the indelible connection of history and memory. Third, the demand to remember runs counter to the impulse to protect the institution and its reputation: the greater the ethical and legal odiousness of an act, the greater the desire to protect the institution and the harder it will be to accomplish the goal of bearing witness. The interaction of these countervailing tendencies admits a range of possibilities: institutions only tangentially involved might be willing to offer more details about the past, and an institution directly responsible for an event of little historical or present impact might try to forget its problematic past. The different qualities identified here each play to some degree a role in the fashioning of the public memory, but before examining the memory work in these key episodes, the history of medical research and the push toward regulating research in the twentieth century must be addressed.

CHAPTER 2

Experiment or Treatment?

HISTORIES OF MEDICAL CARE, RESEARCH,
AND REGULATION

———•◆•———

History and memory are entangled in multiple ways—especially
in bioethics, where truncated versions of history often become
the narrative content of bioethical memory. A number of historical and sociological trends led to the practices of medical research
in the mid-twentieth century that ultimately outraged the collective
conscience, leading to the birth of bioethics and the creation of research
regulation. The horrific actions of American medical researchers in the
twentieth century are not the result of uniquely evil characters. Rather,
they reflect the practice of medicine, both clinical care and research, as
they developed following the Civil War alongside the increased push to
professionalize medicine in the latter half of the nineteenth century.

To better situate the instances of bioethical memory discussed in
the following chapters, this chapter will discuss the history of medicine
in the United States, with special attention given to the relationship
between clinical care and research. While drawing from prior historical

25

research, I will argue that three trends shaped the terrain of medical care and medical research in the middle of the twentieth century: the growth of medicine as a profession shaped by an ethic of benevolent paternalism; the articulation of biopower into *usability* where all bodies had to contribute to the ends of the state; and the perennial blurring of the lines between experiments and therapy existing in medicine since the time of Hippocrates.

The "Birth" of Experimental Medicine

In many ways, experimentation has always been a part of medicine, making any note of its "birth" problematic. As Ruth R. Faden and Tom L. Beauchamp observe, "The practice of research with human subjects is virtually as ancient as medicine itself, but concern about its consequences and about the protection of human subjects is a recent phenomenon."[1] Greek physicians would tinker with medications and see how patients responded to them, in a sense "experimenting" their way toward a person's cure.[2] That impulse persisted in Western medicine through the medieval and Enlightenment eras.[3] Yet those early experimentalist impulses did not lead to generalizable knowledge of medicine or biology as we understand them today, because medicine until the 1860s operated on a principle of "specificity." According to Susan E. Lederer, "physicians prescribed medical therapy that matched the specific characteristics of the individual patient and the social and physical environment of the patient."[4] That impulse was replaced by a growing awareness that medical knowledge about one group could inform treatment of others. That awareness dovetailed with an information explosion in biological and medical sciences in the 1870s. American medical doctors responded to this by calling for medical education to emphasize laboratory techniques and practical clinical encounters.[5] Alongside this recognition came the call from some leaders of the medical community to use hospitals to continue expanding medical knowledge, as well as educating future physicians.[6]

Yet, the experimentation and research implied by the use of hospitals raised concerns for physicians.[7] Harming patients in experiments violated the primary ethic of medicine—the Hippocratic dictum to do no harm. The primary concern was to minimize potential harms and maximize the potential benefits for research participants. There was also some recognition that patients needed to agree to participate: The need for consent mirrors the ethical and legal requirement for nineteenth-century physicians to get consent for medical interventions like surgery. Yet the degree to which consent was sought, or legally required, is unclear. As Lederer notes,

> Patients' consent was a complicated and often ambiguous feature of experimentation, both therapeutic and nontherapeutic. Just as hospital patients served as "clinical material" in the teaching of medical students, they were expected to agree to being part of a trial of a new drug or procedure when their physicians believed that it promised some benefit to them or at least did not harm them.[8]

When physicians conducted research involving the use of standard medical practices, such as blood pressure or temperature readings and reviews of observations noted in medical charts, consent was often bypassed as the potential harm was minimal or nonexistent and the potential benefits for the patient and future patients great. When physicians conducted research that placed patients at risk or had little possible benefit, they were expected to obtain the consent of the patient, but eliciting consent was more about limiting a physician's legal liability than it was an ethical recognition of patient autonomy. Overall, physicians in the late nineteenth century until World War II exercised what Faden and Beauchamp described as an "entrenched Hippocratic authoritarianism" in research and normal medical treatment.[9]

While benevolent paternalism might have assuaged physicians' consciences and satisfied American courts, it would not eliminate all public concern about medical experimentation. During this period, physicians mitigated those concerns by first experimenting on themselves: "The obligation to try a new drug or procedure on oneself (or one's pet) before applying it to patients was an accepted feature of medical research in the mid-nineteenth century. . . . Unwillingness to try a new remedy on oneself or one's family before applying it to patients continued to be a cause for criticism in the late nineteenth century."[10] One of the best-known examples of self-experimentation involved the army's yellow fever experiments in Cuba, led by Walter Reed.[11] Reed and colleagues believed that mosquitoes spread yellow fever. To prove it, two of Reed's colleagues, James Carroll and Jesse Lazear, let themselves be bitten by mosquitoes that had fed on patients with yellow fever. Both men quickly developed yellow fever, and Lazear died from the disease. The surviving members of the team then conducted further experiments involving American soldiers and Spanish emigrants to Cuba. These experiments involved contracts and explicit informed consent, alongside medical care for the yellow fever many contracted (and $100 in gold for Spanish volunteers who developed yellow fever). Practices of self-experimentation helped assuage public concern about medical experimentation by assuring publics that either there was minimal risk, or (as with the yellow fever experiments) that physicians were willing to assume the risk alongside the public. It also allowed researchers to create narratives of scientific martyrs, selflessly risking their lives to forward science and medical care.[12]

This period also saw the first demands for the usability of populations in institutions for the developmentally disabled, orphanages, and prisons —groups not otherwise contributing economically or reproductively to the state. In the 1890s, researchers, including the surgeon general of the United States, tested the efficacy of various vaccines on orphans and developmentally disabled children.[13] In 1911, Hideyo Noguchi, a researcher in New York's Rockefeller Institute for Medical Research, researched a potential skin test for syphilis, and he used patients from across the New York metropolitan area, including hospital patients and forty-six healthy children between the ages of two and eighteen. In 1915, prisoners in Mississippi were used in a study to identify whether poor nutrition was the cause of pellagra, a condition whose symptoms included inflamed skin, diarrhea, sores in the mouth, and eventually dementia: Prisoners who stayed on the poor nutrition diet for six months were offered a pardon by Mississippi's governor Earl Brewer.[14] In 1921, Alfred Hess, along with Mildred Fish and Lester Unger, studied the development of scurvy by withholding orange juice from children at New York City's Home for Hebrew Infants "until the babies developed the small hemorrhages characteristic of the disease" on two occasions.[15] Identifying the cause of various conditions and testing the efficacy of vaccines required large groups of healthy individuals. Individuals in institutions represented to researchers an ideal population, and the sense that all individuals had to contribute to the state in one form or another justified their use.

This is not to say that there was no outcry by the public or qualms on the part of physicians and researchers. The anti-vivisectionist movement in the late nineteenth and early twentieth centuries fought against human experimentation. They saw experimentation on animals and experimentation on humans as a continuum, where "unrestrained experimentation on animals would culminate in the scientific exploitation of vulnerable human beings."[16] Playwright George Bernard Shaw coined the phrase "human guinea pig" in the early twentieth century "to make clear the anti-vivisector's equation of human and animal subjects."[17] Anti-vivisectors saw the work of Noguchi, Hess, and others as emblematic of their concerns, and made these scientists and doctors the focus of their anti-experimentation campaigns.

Similarly, medical researchers had qualms about some of the research being conducted and published. Walter Bradford Cannon of the American Medical Association proposed regulations for research on humans in 1909 and again in 1916, but the leadership of the AMA as well as the broader research community could not come to consensus on any guidelines for research, especially the issue of informed consent.[18] Researchers had difficulty distinguishing between innovative treatment, experiments with a therapeutic outcome (e.g., participation in vaccination trials), and nontherapeutic experiments, and they felt that certain research practices, like collecting urine or blood samples and measuring temperature and blood pressure, were too benign to require formalized consent. They were also concerned about how to acquire consent—such as how much information was required and could patients understand it, and how one mitigates the power imbalance of the doctor-patient relationship to avoid coercion. Physicians and medical researchers could not unravel these issues. Ultimately, these complicated moral and ethical questions were set aside while physicians fought against the efforts to legislate research by anti-vivisectionists and tried to eliminate "quackery"—dubious medical treatments offered by supposed doctors that competed with physicians organized by the AMA.[19]

Despite all the public and technical debate about experimentation, medical research remained unregulated. Even voluntary standards for ethically conducting medical research on people would not be developed until after World War II. Narratives of self-experimentation and medical self-sacrifice, alongside the extraordinary successes of medicine and medical research, vouchsafed for the status quo. Anti-vivisectionists and their concerns were eventually marginalized by the start of World War II. American researchers and the American public were content to trust individual physicians and their judgment of the best course of action for patients and research participants.

Medical Research during and after World War II

World War II intensified the trends of earlier medical research.[20] Benevolent paternalism, the drive to usability, and the confusion of therapy and research continued. These concerns became more prominent as medical research burgeoned during the war and after the Nazi medical atrocities were revealed. During the war, medical research was overseen by the Committee on Medical Research (CMR), established in the summer of 1941.[21] The CMR organized contracts with universities to conduct medical research, and by the end of the war, it had funded 593 contracts worth $24 million that involved the work of more than five thousand investigators.[22] The accomplishments of the CMR were impressive. Penicillin was refined and distributed to the European and Pacific Theaters, as well as hospitals in the United States.[23] Other accomplishments included developing gamma globulin (a treatment for hepatitis), blood transfusion and blood substitutes, other treatments for dysentery and malaria, and the production of insecticides to control mosquitoes and other pests.[24] Much of the disease research in World War II repeated the most problematic aspects of pre–World War II research. For example, studies on dysentery and influenza used patients in institutions for the developmentally disabled, and research on malaria used prisoners as research subjects.[25] Wartime necessity reinforced the need to render all bodies useful. The war made experimentation "a patriotic necessity for all Americans. Men, women, and children were pressed into service as research subjects as researchers joined the war efforts . . . moral qualms about using these populations [i.e., developmentally disabled, orphans, and prisoners] in nontherapeutic studies faded in the harsh light of wartime necessity."[26] Researchers, the government, and the public all saw the success of medical research and considered the costs acceptable, to the degree that they knew the costs.

The federal government continued funding and providing intellectual direction to medical research after the war. This was part of the broader vision for American investment in basic science articulated by Vannevar Bush in a report titled *Science, the Endless Frontier.*[27] Medical research was primarily supported by the National Institutes of Health (NIH), but additional research (primarily focused on understanding the effects of radiation) was supported by the Atomic Energy Commission, the Department of Defense, and the Department of Energy.[28]

THE NUREMBERG CODE

While the American research enterprise expanded, some politicians, lawyers, and physicians grappled anew with the ethics of medical research in light of the Nuremberg trial of Nazi physicians who experimented on people in concentration camps. While they were not the first example of willfully harmful research in medical history, "the Nazi experiments were in many respects unprecedented in the extensiveness and extremity of the harm and suffering to which they knowingly exposed their victims."[29] Experiments included exploring "the effects of ingesting poisons, intravenous injections of gasoline, immersion in ice water . . . infection with epidemic jaundice and spotted fever virus," among others.[30] An American military tribunal tried the Nazi physicians. The trial ran from December 9, 1946, to August 19, 1947, and in their verdict against the physicians, the military tribunal articulated a set of ten standards for medical experimentation. They included requirements for informed and voluntary consent, prior experimentation on animals, and a balancing of risks to participants and potential benefits for the participants and society.[31]

Yet, the impact of the Nuremberg Code on American research practices was uneven at best. The trials and the code did lead to the creation of several policy documents in the United States. In December 1946, as a result of reports from consultants to the Nuremberg prosecutors, the American Medical Association revised its code of ethics to require voluntary consent of research participants.[32] While the rules were published and were disseminated to most American physicians, "these rules were not published prominently; they were set in small type along with a variety of other miscellaneous business items. . . . Only an exceptionally diligent member [of the AMA], or one with a special interest in medical ethics, is likely to have located this item."[33] In 1947, the Atomic Energy Commission's general manager created a series of statements outlining requirements that university contractors solicit verbal consent from participants, but the "statements were not routinely communicated in response to requests for guidance from non-AEC researchers."[34] Finally, in 1953, Department of Defense secretary Charles Wilson established that the Nuremberg Code would be the operating ethical policy for DOD research; but the memorandum outlining this policy was classified top secret and not circulated widely, limiting its impact.[35]

At roughly the same time, the NIH's Clinical Center, a 500-bed research hospital on the NIH's Bethesda campus, adopted a policy for research on human participants.[36] The policy required at least verbal consent from all research participants and "written consent from healthy subjects and from only certain patient-subjects," as well as prior review of research protocols by other physicians and researchers at the Clinical Center.[37] While the NIH had participated in the DOD's deliberations over human subjects,[38] the extent to which the Nuremberg Code influenced NIH policy is not clear. Charles McCarthy argues that the policy was rooted in changes "in the appreciation of ethical issues in medical research" without specifying the basis for those changes.[39] Regardless of the impetus, the NIH Clinical Center developed a policy that mirrored many of the principles of the Nuremberg Code. Yet, that policy was limited to the Clinical Center, not all NIH-funded research, and it never included clear standards for what researchers needed to disclose to participants about risks and benefits, details of procedures, etc.[40]

Policies based on the principles of the Nuremberg Code were developed by many of the agencies involved in human subjects research, but those policies were not disseminated widely to the researchers who needed to implement them. Even if the policies had been disseminated, it is not clear what influence they would have had with researchers and funding agencies. First, issues of usability influenced the degree to which the federal government enforced its existing policies, especially in the context of DOD research. For example, since the time of Walter Reed, research by the armed services had a tradition of informed consent, but as the Advisory Committee on Human Radiation Experiments (ACHRE) noted, the imposition of ethical limits on researchers "depended on the nature of its [DOD's] interest in the research being done."[41] In other words, the needs of the state determined whether ethical considerations trumped usability.

Second, American medical researchers did not see the Nuremberg Code and its principles as relevant to their activities. David Rothman states that American researchers viewed the Nazi physicians as "Nazis first and last; by definition, nothing they did, and no code drawn up in response to them, was relevant to the United States."[42] Similarly, Allan M. Brandt and Lara Freidenfels argued that in the immediate aftermath of World War II, "researchers cited Nazi science as an example of the potential abuses of government oversight and control."[43] In other words, outside forces—the government and Nazis—produced the experiments in the Nazi concentration camps, not medical researchers directly.

Third, concerns about maintaining the sanctity of the doctor-patient relationship and ongoing confusion of clinical treatment with research impacted how researchers and funding agencies understood research regulation policies. During the period from 1946 through the following decade, medical researchers and the government agencies funding research viewed research through the lens of the doctor-patient relationship, where "patient trust and medical beneficence were viewed as the unshakeable moral foundations on which meaningful interactions between professional healers and the sick should be built."[44] The paternalistic legacy of Hippocrates guaranteed that judgments of beneficence were the purview of the individual physician: If a physician believed a course of treatment was beneficial and risks trivial, there was no pressing need to acquire consent from patients or research participants. Because a great deal of medical research involved people who were already ill, physicians and many other groups believed "that the researcher-subject relationship was identical to the doctor-patient relationship."[45] Since the doctor-patient relationship was a *private* one, government funding agencies were leery of interfering with it, and physician-researchers would regularly argue that requiring consent, especially written consent, violated their relationship with patient-subjects.[46] Overall, the confusion of research and treatment within the context of the paternalistic doctor-patient relationship, along with the state's willingness to use some people to further research of military and medical interest, was the context of normal medical research for most of the twentieth century. This created the space for medicine to go obviously and publicly wrong in the 1960s.

THE PUSH FOR RESEARCH REGULATION

Starting in the 1960s, politicians, philosophers, and the lay public generally became concerned about medical practice, especially medical research practices. Scholars offer two overlapping reasons for this change.[47] First, the protest movements of the 1960s and 1970s—civil rights, women's rights, LGBT rights, the consumer movement, etc.—focused attention on individual rights, choice, and autonomy, among other broader issues, and these movements often included concerns about health care and medicine. Second, these movements also encouraged a distrust of authority and paternalism, which were the cornerstones of medical practice. The demand to respect individual patients and their choices, along with the distrust of authority were crystallized by a series of scandals.

In 1961, American trust in medicine and the "miracles" medical research provided were shaken by the thalidomide scandal.[48] Doctors had prescribed the sedative thalidomide to countless pregnant women in Canada, across Europe, and to a lesser degree in the United States. Thalidomide produced countless birth defects, primarily children born with missing or deformed limbs. According to ACHRE, the thalidomide disaster was widely covered by the media, especially television, and "the visual impact of these babies stunned viewers and caused Americans to question the protections afforded those receiving investigational agents [i.e., experimental drugs and medical treatments]."[49] The scandal led Congress to empower the Food and Drug Administration to test new medications for safety and efficacy, and also to require informed consent for individuals involved in testing the new drugs.

In 1963, one of the first notorious cases of medical research in the post–World War II era came to light, the Jewish Chronic Disease Hospital (JCDH) cancer study. Dr. Chester M. Southam led this study where twenty-two patients at the JCDH in Brooklyn, New York, were injected with live cancer cells. According to Faden and Beauchamp, "Southam had convinced [JCDH medical director Emmanuel E.] Mandel that although the research was entirely nontherapeutic, it was routine to do such research without consent."[50] Most of the patients were poor, and some of them were senile or had dementia. Even those patients who could have given informed consent were not told they would be injected with cancer cells "because to do so might agitate them unnecessarily."[51] Three junior physicians at the hospital refused to participate in the study and resigned a few weeks after the study was initiated without them.[52] As news of the research and the resignation of the three residents percolated

through the hospital and New York medical community, medical authorities tried to contain and downplay the event until William E. Hyman,
a lawyer and JCDH cofounder and board member, sued the hospital to
get details from internal committees about the research.[53] Amidst the
hostile public reaction to revelations of the study, the New York State
Board of Regents "suspended the licenses of Drs. Mandel and Southam,
but subsequently stayed the suspension and placed the physicians on
probation for one year."[54] Medical researchers rallied around Southam;
in fact, a few years later, they elected him president of the American Association for Cancer Research.[55] Overall, this incident highlights medical
paternalism in Southam and Mandel's reliance on Southam's judgment
of risk alone, ignoring oversight committees and the concerns of junior
colleagues, as well as the willingness to render indigent elderly patients
with dementia usable for the nation-state through research.

While medical researchers generally rallied around Southam and
defended their professional prerogatives to determine the course of research, leaders of medical research, especially NIH director James Shannon, were disturbed by the details of Southam's research and the negative
public reaction to it. As a result, Shannon pushed for the development
of guidelines for clinical research that recognized for the first time that
the researcher-participant relationship differed substantially from the
doctor-patient relationship.[56] Shannon's efforts led to the creation of a
Public Health Service (PHS) policy published in 1966 that recognized
that "patient-subjects, like healthy subjects, should be included in the
consent provisions for federally sponsored human experimentation."[57]
The PHS tried to balance federal regulation and local control of research.
As a result, "the new rules were neither as intrusive as some investigators
feared nor as protective as some advocates preferred."[58]

While the NIH and PHS were developing new standards for research, Henry Beecher, an anesthesiologist from Harvard, published
what is considered the most important medical publication on medical
ethics in the mid-twentieth century.[59] Beecher published an account of
twenty-two anonymized cases of medical research that he felt "endan-
gered the health and well-being of subjects without their knowledge or

approval."[60] The research was conducted at prominent medical institutions: "Four came from Harvard Medical School, three from the NIH Clinical Center, and the rest from other prominent institutions."[61] To help disseminate his findings and his concerns, Beecher distributed an earlier version of the article to journalists in 1965, but refused to give interviews: "This was the beginning of Beecher's strategy of speaking directly in the medical literature only, but making sure that the public heard about his criticisms second-hand. That way, he gave the appearance that he was prompting a discussion within the medical profession, which the public happened to be observing, rather than inviting the public to join the discussion."[62] For all his concern about unethical research, Beecher's suggested course of action still reinforced the professional prerogatives of medical researchers. He was opposed to outside regulation and ethical codes, including the Nuremberg Code. He doubted "the ability of a formal code of ethics to shape researchers' behavior" and called for researchers to be more responsible in their conduct of research.[63]

One of the twenty-two studies identified by Beecher was Saul Krugman's study of hepatitis at the Willowbrook State School.[64] Yet, while the study was easily identified from Beecher's description despite his attempt to anonymize it, the study did not receive much attention in 1966. The study finally became notorious after Beecher offered an expanded discussion of it in his 1970 book and after the publication in *The Lancet* of criticism by Stephen Goldby.[65] This debate and the research continued until the public outrage about conditions at the school started the process of the school's closure in 1972.

Then, in 1972, alongside the controversies over the Willowbrook hepatitis study, there was the public revelation of the Tuskegee Syphilis Study. Despite the PHS creating guidelines for research in 1966, the study had continued. Individuals, like Henry Beecher and Jay Katz, who had been concerned about informed consent in medical research missed the study in their canvass of medical publications for questionable research.[66] Public revelation of the study brought outrage, and in the face of that outrage, the Department of Health, Education, and Welfare (DHEW) created the Tuskegee Syphilis Study Ad Hoc Advisory

Panel, consisting of nine men and women from a range of professions, of whom five were black and four were white.[67] Their purpose was "to review the study as well as the Department's policies and procedures for the protection of human subjects in general."[68] The panel declared that the study should be terminated at once, the men remaining in the study should receive all health care necessary to treat disabilities that resulted from their participation, and better protections for human subjects were needed in all DHEW research, which included the work of the NIH and the PHS.[69]

Other stories of dubious medical research percolated through medical and public discourse, like the Cincinnati Whole Body Radiation (WBS) study, but most of those received substantially less attention at the time.[70] These three scandals—JCDH, Willowbrook, and Tuskegee—received the most attention, and it was Tuskegee that in many ways guaranteed congressional action. The earliest attempts at congressional oversight of research occurred in 1968. Walter Mondale introduced a bill for a Commission on Health, Science, and Society.[71] The bill faced "unbending opposition" from medical researchers who "fought doggedly to maintain their authority over all medical matters."[72] The opposition was so virulent that it left Mondale "disgusted" with medical practitioners, and he continued fighting for research regulation with little success through 1973.[73] His quest was successful after he was joined by Senator Edward Kennedy. Kennedy chaired the hearings on the syphilis study at Tuskegee. The hearing featured testimony from men in the study, their attorney Fred Gray, and members of the DHEW Ad Hoc Panel.[74] David Rothman argues, "Kennedy, more artfully than Mondale earlier, structured the hearings to demonstrate the need for outside intervention."[75] During these hearings and later, Kennedy would repeatedly invoke "the great scandals in human experimentation—Willowbrook, Tuskegee, Brooklyn Jewish Chronic Disease Hospital."[76] Kennedy's efforts, along with Mondale's, led to the successful passage of the National Research Act in 1974: It established a National Commission that "did pioneering work as it addressed issues of autonomy, informed consent, and third-party permission, particularly in relation to research involving vulnerable subjects such as prisoners, children, and people with cognitive disabilities."[77] While the commission produced multiple reports, perhaps the most important is the Belmont Report, which defined the fundamental values that should guide the ethical conduct of research. The values and processes of risk-benefit calculation and informed consent have shaped research regulation in the United States since 1981.

Conclusion

History and the various forms of public memory are entangled. This especially holds true for bioethics, where, as Susan Reverby observed, truncated versions of various histories become bioethical memories in the space of the classroom. Memory and history in bioethics converge; the most important events of the mid-twentieth century—the scandalous research that produced public outrage and medical indifference—become the milestones of memory. As Susan Reverby notes, the JCDH cancer study, Willowbrook hepatitis study, and the Tuskegee syphilis study formed the "'holy trinity' of American horror stories of research."[78] Historically and in memory narratives, they serve as the impetus for regulating medical research in the United States.

Along with this convergence around major mid-twentieth-century events, there are divergences and gaps as well. The story of medical research in America arguably begins at the close of the Civil War as changing medical philosophies and increasing professionalization made research a logical adjunct to treatment. Yet American medicine and medical research maintained its Hippocratic authoritarianism, the benevolent paternalism that gave the individual judgment of physicians and physician-researchers primacy. While medical professionals recognized a role for some type of patient consent in their various clinical and research practices, that consent often looked nothing like the informed consent practiced today and was subordinated to medical judgments of acceptable risks. This paternalism is well-recognized in the histories of medicine and bioethics, but it appears rarely in bioethics training. For example, CITI training (Collaborative Institutional Training Initiative) mentions that research occurred in the late nineteenth century but dates concerns about research ethics to the Nuremberg trials, and it does not mention paternalism at all.[79] Similarly, while issues of usability and the impact of medical professionalism appear in various medical histories, they do not appear at all in memory products from the bioethics classroom. The impact of professionalism and the drive to protect the medical authority and the reputation of medical research plays a major role in the reaction of researchers to the initial congressional attempts at oversight. It also, as we will see, encourages the minimal remembrance and forgetting that haunts bioethical memory, especially in the case of the Cincinnati WBS study.

While elements of this bioethics history are conspicuously absent from memory in the classroom, some of those elements appear more prominently in public memorials that constitute bioethical memory. Key moments in this history, as it appears in public, differ as well. For example, there is no public memorial to the Jewish Chronic Disease Hospital study. The Cincinnati WBS study, which is mentioned by David Rothman, does not play a prominent role in histories of medical regulation but does have a monument dedicated to it. Bioethical memory as it appears in classrooms differs from bioethical memory as it appears in public remembrance. Yet, these different facets of bioethical memory draw from the same broad history and can influence each other. To see the interaction of the identities, affective investments, and other priorities of medical professionals and other groups play out in public instances of bioethical memory, we now turn to an examination of the museums and memorials, starting with the museums dedicated to the syphilis study conducted in Tuskegee, Alabama, and the surrounding county.

PART 2

Cases of Bioethical Memory
and Minimal Remembrance

———•———

CHAPTER 3

Lawsuits and Legacies

COMPETING MEMORIALIZATIONS
OF THE TUSKEGEE SYPHILIS STUDY

———•◆•———

On July 26, 1972, Jean Heller of the Associated Press broke the story of the Tuskegee Syphilis Study, the U.S. Public Health Service (PHS)–run observation of six hundred African American men in rural Macon County, Alabama, of whom four hundred had latent stage syphilis.[1] The men were told they had "bad blood," a term used to describe a host of ailments ranging from anemia to syphilis. They were kept in the Study through incentives like free meals, rides into Tuskegee, Alabama—the county seat of Macon County and home to the Tuskegee Institute—and burial insurance. They were also told that pink baby aspirin and iron tonics they received, along with a painful spinal tap procedure conducted when the Study opened, were "treatments" for their bad blood. The deceptions were intended both to keep the men in the Study throughout their lives and to prevent them from seeking actual treatment, including the penicillin that became available in the mid-1940s.[2] The Study ran for forty years, and only a handful of medical researchers ever experienced a sense of the *unheimlich* that led them to question the ethics of the research. Ultimately, as one PHS official noted, "nothing learned will ever prevent, find, or cure a single case of infectious syphilis."[3]

The public disclosure of the Study led to a welter of rhetorical activity. As Susan Reverby observes, it generated "rumors, historical monographs, videos, documentaries, plays, poems, music, a movie, photomontages, a surgeon general's nomination hearings, a presidential apology, a common topic for IRB training, new memorials, and a National Bioethics Institute."[4] The United States Public Health Service's Study of Untreated Syphilis became transformed in public discourse into the "Tuskegee Syphilis Study," or more often just "Tuskegee."[5] Thomas and Quinn's conclusion is apt: "Today, the Tuskegee Study transcends its historical time and geographical context to emerge as a metaphor for racism in research."[6] Bioethicists and historians have alternately described Tuskegee as a myth, metaphor, allegory, narrative, and as a memory.[7]

Susan Reverby's work has examined a wide range of the discourses around Tuskegee within the frame of "cultural memory" and highlights how the "facts" and "fictions" found there are productive of attitudes toward medical research, government-funded research, race, and racism. One area not fully addressed by Reverby and others is the material rhetorics and "public memory" developed in museums dedicated to the Study—the Tuskegee History Center and the Tuskegee University Legacy Museum.[8] Both sites proffer public memories of what is considered the greatest medical and bioethical abuse in the United States. They can both be found in Tuskegee, just a short drive from one another. This highlights two of the theoretical commonplaces in memory scholarship: the importance of place and the competition between different partial memories of an event.

In what follows, I argue that the Tuskegee History Center and the Legacy Museum offer distinct and competing visions of the Tuskegee Syphilis Study. The History Center encourages visitors to witness the details of the Study and identify themselves as part of a people defined by the law and civil rights. It emphasizes the successful lawsuit against the U.S. government by the Study survivors, placing the Study within a vision of the civil rights movement, defined as a series of successful litigation efforts in the 1950s and early 1960s. The Legacy Museum recuperates the legacy of Tuskegee Institute and the city of Tuskegee by emphasizing the area's contribution to African American welfare through research and education and by renaming the Study as the "United States Public Health Service Study of Untreated Syphilis in the Male Negro, 1932–1972." In doing so, the Legacy Museum positions visitors as witnesses to the Institute's struggles against (medical) racism. Before examining the two museums, I consider the extant memories of Tuskegee circulating in a variety of discursive arenas.

Extant Memories of Tuskegee

The United States Study of Untreated Syphilis in the Negro Male—as the Study was originally named—ran from 1932 to 1972, a period of massive change in the United States that included the Depression, World War II, and the civil rights movement. Out of this rich, convoluted, and sometimes obscured history, many memories could be crafted; yet a relatively coherent narrative has emerged. As Reverby observes, "Memory [of the Study] brings the research community and the public *together,* as narratives of ethics and memories of oppression became interlocked."[9] Yet, within that singular narrative, medical researchers (especially bioethicists) and the general public each select and deflect different aspects of the Study's history in their memory making, producing three broad configurations of memory: memories of medical research, memories of race and racism, and a partially suppressed memory of institutional shame that challenges how the Study is named.

MEMORIES OF MEDICAL RESEARCH

The work of bioethicists is responsible in many ways for the existence of public memory of Tuskegee. "Bioethicists kept knowledge of the Study alive in research publications and teaching," argues Susan Reverby, "but only in narrow ways."[10] The meaning of Tuskegee is relatively clear: "Tuskegee is a red flag for bioethics."[11] As Reverby argues, "The story [of Tuskegee] would become one of the failures of researchers to consider informed consent and of the callous disregard for the vulnerable."[12] This failure of oversight became a justification for creating the regulatory tools to guarantee informed consent and protect the vulnerable. This story constitutes audiences as witnesses to the limits of the paternalism in post-Flexner medicine where the Hippocratic Oath acted as the sole moral compass. The considered judgment of the physician was supposed to protect those vulnerable individuals enrolled in research from undue harm, and it failed miserably. Memories of Tuskegee (and the other American research stories) became a way for physicians to recognize the ethical limits of how medical research used to be performed. This recognition is then channeled by the narrative into support for Belmont Report values and the systems of research protection put into place to realize those values.

Yet this version of Tuskegee downplays the role of race in medical thinking, complicating attempts at reforming medical research. By framing the issue as one of "vulnerability," the bioethics memory "provided a way to say that race matters and then to never really interrogate in what ways."[13] Bioethicists knew that segregation and racial discrimination left the men "vulnerable," but foregrounding "vulnerability" deflected considerations of racial injustice while also allowing the African American men of Tuskegee, Alabama, to be compared to mentally handicapped children on Staten Island and elderly Jewish patients in Brooklyn, New York. Such a move was functionally important for justifying research regulation with a broad reach, but it left the racist roots of black "vulnerability" unaddressed.

Additionally, the placement of the story, both in relation to other research and in terms of geography, makes it challenging for many medical researchers to identify with the narrative. Tuskegee is the first—chronologically and in perceived magnitude—of *America*'s research crimes, but it is not the first crime mentioned in bioethics's origin story. That dubious honor goes to the Nuremberg trials of Nazi doctors for medical experiments conducted in concentration camps. Typically, these narratives begin in Germany and then cross the Atlantic to land in Alabama: "When the litany went directly from Nazis to Tuskegee, the details of the study entered a historical fog. Alabama became a prison, the men were concentration camp victims, and the PHS morphed into Nazis."[14] The linkage of the PHS researchers in Alabama with Nazi doctors distances contemporary medical researchers from Tuskegee and the racism that enabled the Study.[15] It also encourages viewing the men in the Study as a monolithic and abject group: The men in the Study are framed as vulnerable because they were Depression-era, illiterate, black sharecroppers, and "the differing occupational, educational, and personal identities of the men are erased as they become, as a group, every Southern black man, available as symbols of revictimization."[16] The memory produced about Tuskegee centers images of Depression-era black sharecroppers to emphasize vulnerability while distancing contemporary researchers from the research practices of the PHS during the Study and also ironically obscuring issues of race.

LAY MEMORIES OF RACE AND RACISM

Tuskegee also became a vehicle for a memory of racism that exceeds the boundaries of medical research. Reverby observes, "It [Tuskegee] has gained nearly as much power as slavery and lynching to define the refusal to consider African Americans as rights-bearing citizens."[17] Here, the concern is not about developing reflection on medical research practice. Instead, the goal is to create *philia* through anger and outrage at the history of injustices against African Americans.

This articulation of public memory has its roots in events in the 1970s, specifically the lawsuit by civil rights attorney Fred Gray on behalf of the men in the Study and their families. In July 1973, Gray, who had first risen to national prominence for serving as an attorney for Rosa Parks and Martin Luther King Jr. during the Montgomery Bus Boycott, filed a $1.8 billion class action suit against the United

States government, the Department of Health Education and Welfare (now the Department of Health and Human Services), the U.S. Public Health Service, the Centers for Disease Control (CDC), the State of Alabama, the Alabama State Board of Health, the Milbank Fund (which had provided the burial insurance used as an incentive to keep men in the Study), the heads of all the federal and state agencies involved, and three individual PHS officers.[18] The case was ultimately settled out of court in December 1974.[19]

Gray framed his case around racial discrimination and victimization. The Ninth, Thirteenth, and Fourteenth Amendments featured prominently in Gray's original filings.[20] He argued that "participants were poor, Southern, rural, African Americans," "no white persons were solicited and used for the study," and "those selected were used in a program of controlled genocide solely because of their race and color."[21] These legal strategies meant that "no predominately black institution was named in the suit . . . [and] all the individually named defendants were white."[22] The lawsuit and the media reports of it fashioned "a black-and-white story in which justice was to be found in legal proceeding through financial compensation to a victimized group."[23] Reportage on the Study and Gray's lawsuit reflected and amplified the framing of the experiment as an embodiment of racism: "As the story then spun out, the men became every southern black man, their individuality lost, and the crimes against them a measure of the depth of public racism."[24]

Over the years, the story exceeded the frame of research to become incorporated into larger narratives of black vulnerability and official malevolence. Stories in the 1980s framing events as diverse as the appearance of crack cocaine, the existence of HIV/AIDS, and the use of needle exchange programs would include mention of Tuskegee as proof that the government was capable of long-running conspiracies against African Americans.[25] Tuskegee was also invoked by filmmaker Spike Lee to explain federal responses to Hurricane Katrina.[26] In these examples, references to Tuskegee constitute audiences as witnesses to racism in multiple contexts.

MEMORY OF DISGRACE AND SHAME

In addition to the bioethical memory and the memory of race and racism, there is an additional memory of the Tuskegee Syphilis Study as the source of shame for Macon County, Alabama. Like memories that tie the Study into broader narratives of race and racism, this strand of memory draws from a broader history as well: It amplifies criticism of Booker T. Washington—the first principal of the Tuskegee Institute—and the Tuskegee Institute's approach to black empowerment in the twentieth century. It highlights Washington's 1895 Cotton States and International Exhibition speech in Atlanta, Georgia. In that speech, he argued for modest attempts at black self-improvement and discarded Reconstruction-era attempts at equality with his claim that "in all things that are purely social, we can be as separate as the fingers, yet one as the hand in all things essential to mutual progress."[27] Washington's approach to racial uplift and empowerment also had overt class biases, as "he tried to create what came to be called 'a New Negro,' in a break from the perceived 'stereotypes' of licentiousness and 'minstrelsy.'"[28] This led to subsequent criticism, like that of W. E. B. Du Bois in 1904.[29] One of the most vivid critiques of the Tuskegee Institute—and by implication, Booker T. Washington—as perpetuators of a classism and paternalism in their program of racial uplift is found in Ralph Ellison's *Invisible Man*. The book's narrator attends an all-black college modeled on the Tuskegee Institute. He is expelled by its principal, Dr. Bledsoe (a stand-in for Tuskegee's second principal, Robert Moton), after allowing a white trustee to see the poverty of rural black life off the campus. Dr. Bledsoe goes so far as to sabotage the narrator's search for a job in New York City, sacrificing the narrator to Bledsoe's vision of racial betterment.[30]

While broader political issues influence the degree to which memory implicates the Institute in the Study, there is evidence that some prominent members of the Institute, its John A. Andrews Hospital, and the nearby African American–run veterans hospital *did* know about and support it. The doctors from the Public Health Service reached out to Robert Moton and to the head of the Tuskegee Institute's hospital, Eugene Dibble, on multiple occasions to get the Institute's support for the Study.[31] According to James Jones, the participation of the Tuskegee Institute was vital: "The Institute's cooperation would permit the study to go forward without arousing the fears and suspicions of private physicians. The participation of black physicians would also help secure the cooperation of subjects for the experiment, for the Tuskegee Institute commanded trust and respect among the black population of Macon County."[32] Because much of the information about what Tuskegee Institute officials knew comes from the PHS, accounts vary in the degree to which they held Tuskegee officials culpable. Jones is strident in his denunciation: "Dr. Moton and Dr. Dibble both knew that black men alone would be studied. . . . The objective of whites was not to deceive [middle class] blacks but to make it easier for them to engage in self-deceit."[33] In his account of the Study and the subsequent lawsuit, Fred Gray is more demure: "There were a few doctors connected with John A. Andrew Memorial Hospital and the Veterans Administration Medical Center in Tuskegee who had some knowledge of the program."[34]

Historical accounts indicate that the leadership of the Tuskegee Institute were aware of the initial plans for the Study in 1932, although the full depth of their knowledge is unclear. Nonetheless, the insinuation that the university was complicit in the Study and in harming the African American residents of the county did circulate through contemporaneous as well as historical discourse. In an article in *Ebony* magazine published shortly after the Study became public, pointed remarks indicting the Institute appear frequently in the captions of photographs. The photograph of Tuskegee's mayor Johnny Ford includes the remark "I was shocked to realize lives had been lost and damaged just for experimental purposes. But what I am really concerned about is the way the image of the city of Tuskegee has been marred."[35] Much of the article consists of an interview with Charlie Pollard, the lead plaintiff in the Study lawsuit. It closes with a picture of Pollard. The caption reads, "Pausing at statue of Booker T. Washington on Tuskegee Institute campus, Pollard seems to be reflecting about campus' academic face and town's syphilis humiliation."[36] The caption is marvelously ambiguous. On the one hand, it might be an attempt to provide context about the impact of the Study on the region: The town is humiliated while the Institute's reputation for working on behalf of African Americans locally and nationally remains unchanged. On the other hand, it can just as equally be an indictment of the policies and the practices of the Institute as well as the Study. Finally, it resonates with Ellison's novel and the scene where the narrator stands in front of a similar statue, debating whether the founder/Washington is lifting the veil or lowering it over the face of the slave.[37]

The insinuation of complicity can equally be a reaction to Washington's politics or a reaction to historical accounts of the Study, but regardless of the motivation, these insinuations were challenged in 1996. The Syphilis Study Committee, a group of academics alongside community activists and officials from Macon County, started a campaign for a federal apology for the Study. Their call for a federal apology highlighted the issue of shame and the reputational harm done to the Institute/ university. They argued,

> Because the name of the study points to Tuskegee Institute (now Tuskegee University) rather than the United States Public Health Service, it clouds the funding and responsibility for the Study. Although facilities and staff of the Tuskegee Institute were involved, primary direction came from the government under the auspices of the USPHS. The notoriety of the Study obscures the achievements of the Tuskegee Institute in improving the health care of African Americans.[38]

For the committee, the name of the Study associates it with the Institute and university rather than the town, and it also implies that the Study was started or managed by Tuskegee Institute rather than merely occurring in the environs of Tuskegee. The claim was compelling enough that Bill Clinton included it in his apology on behalf of the nation for the Study, calling it "the study done in Tuskegee" and saying, "To Macon County, to Tuskegee, to the doctors who have been wrongly associated with the events there, you have our apology as well."[39]

A Tale of Two Museums

The United States PHS (Tuskegee) Syphilis Study has been remembered in multiple ways. These various performances of memory can be divided into three groups—memories associated with medical research and bioethics, memories centered on race and racism, and a memory of the Study as a mark of shame for the Tuskegee Institute. These performances constitute the memoryscape, the conceptual background, that visitors might bring as they encounter the two museums dedicated to the Study in Tuskegee, Alabama. Each museum reflects a different performance of memory. The Tuskegee History Center, founded by lawyer Fred Gray and the living survivors of the Study in 1999, tells a story that positions legal action and the survivors' lawsuit as the key to understanding the region and the larger civil rights movement, while the Legacy Museum works to recover different "legacies" that can be imputed to racism, the Tuskegee Institute, and the Clinton apology, all while never naming or discussing the Study in detail.

THE TUSKEGEE HISTORY CENTER

The Tuskegee History Center is a regional museum that frames the Study as a pivotal moment in the area's history. The public memory of Macon County and the Study that the center articulates depicts events in the region through a legal and civil rights frame. It remembers the area and its history through the lens of an idealized circa-1950s civil rights movement, exemplified by the legal maneuvers associated with Martin Luther King Jr.'s nonviolent protests. This narrative then is also biographical: The center's founder, Fred Gray Sr., was the lawyer for Rosa Parks during the Montgomery Bus boycott, as well as the lead litigator in countless voting rights and desegregation cases.[40] Visitors are called to witness this civil rights history and biography and experience philia as a community characterized by the legal legacy of Macon County.

The center is located in an old bank. It consists of an entrance foyer, the exhibit space (which takes up the majority of the space), and a small

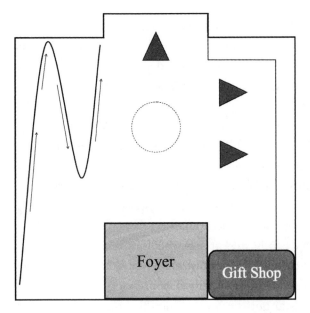

Figure 1. The layout of the Tuskegee History Center. The exhibit space is divided into three sections outlining, respectively, the history of the region, details about the Study, and details about the civil rights movement.

gift shop (see figure 1). From the outset, the center mobilizes the diffuse nature of public memory texts by recognizing the multitude of other memory sites that might be read alongside the museum, while establishing Tuskegee and Macon County as central to that diffuse text. In the foyer, a stand on the right wall has maps and brochures about points of interest in Tuskegee and Macon County, including the Tuskegee Airmen National Historic Site, the Tuskegee Institute National Historic Site, and the Legacy Museum. On the left is a stand with brochures, etc., for sites of interest in Alabama. On the floor, picked out in tile, is the outline of Macon County with the city of Tuskegee noted by a diamond-shaped piece of tile. The center indicates that Tuskegee and Macon County have much to offer visitors, and it also emphasizes the centrality of the county and town to regional and American history.

The exhibit space is divided into three sections one moves through sequentially. The first section covers the history of the area, from the age of the dinosaurs through World War II. This section is organized in a linear, chronological pattern: movement forward past the displays takes one forward in time. While similar to many regional history museums, this section of the exhibit space calls visitors to witness the roles and history of *multiple* cultures and ethnic groups. This emphasis actually begins in the entrance, where visitors see a sculpture depicting three faces that represent the three ethnic groups (from back to front and left to right: Native American, African American, and European American) that the center identifies as the contributors to the history of Macon County, allowing for identification and affiliation from many racial-ethnic viewpoints. The second section is devoted solely to the Tuskegee Syphilis Experiment and the survivors' lawsuit against the federal government. This section is open, with the majority of the space dominated by a marble marker set into the floor. The marker contains the names of all the men who were in the Study, and at its center in a larger font appears the name of their court case, *Charlie W. Pollard et al., v. United States of America et al.* Behind this, located at the back of the exhibit space, is a three-sided display providing details about the Study. The third section is devoted to the civil rights movement, which is framed as a series of legal actions and issues. Two three-sided displays stand equidistant from each other in the middle of this third section, and a timeline of political issues and legal cases runs along the wall under the banner "Macon County, Tuskegee Institute, the City of Tuskegee, played a major role in civil rights . . . —Atty. Fred Gray."

The overall organization of the center is notable for three reasons. First, to move away from the past, which includes slavery, genocide, Jim Crow, the Civil War, etc., into an era of civil rights one must literally cross over the survivors' lawsuit. The lawsuit over the Study literally is the center of the museum. It also stands symbolically as the crux of the region's history and the identities crafted for visitors. The details of the Study, while important, are materially and symbolically the backdrop to the lawsuit. Second, crossing over the lawsuit involves a decisive break in the museum's structure. The first section of the museum is organized chronologically, but the chronological continuity is broken after the first section. The *Pollard et al.* lawsuit was filed in 1973 and settled out of court in 1974, but many of the issues addressed in the third part of the exhibit space predate the lawsuit by decades. The organization of the second and third sections also breaks from the linear construction of the displays and exhibits: they use many freestanding, three-sided displays in which the text makes frequent use of present-perfect, past-perfect, and past-perfect-progressive tenses, alongside some past-tense constructions. Although the specific events mentioned occurred in the past, discursively and materially these sections imply that the action of civil rights is ongoing, and individuals are encouraged to witness and be affiliated with it.

Third, the positioning of the lawsuit is symbolically transformative of themes developed in the first part of the museum. The first section of the center emphasizes the contributions of multiple cultures, the educational efforts in Macon County, and medical racism. African American and Native American people receive considerable attention. Descriptions of the Creek Indians who lived in the region emphasize the role of women in the Creek political and community life. A brief text titled "Creeks and Africans" describes the interactions of the two groups, including positive elements like intermarriage and mixed communities as well as negative elements such as the Creek participation in the slave trade and African Americans' aid in the genocide of Native Americans. While there are positive descriptions of European Americans, the majority of the material in the opening section describes how European Americans introduced smallpox to the Americas and instituted the slave trade. In describing the removal of the Indians from Alabama, European American perfidy is emphasized alongside the plight of the Creek Indians and those African Americans who lived among them. After the removal of the Native American peoples, the history displays spend about equal time describing European Americans and African Americans in the antebellum era through the Second World War.

Education plays a prominent role in the history displays from the antebellum period forward. As the first part of the exhibit opens onto the space where the lawsuit marker is located, the displays describe Tuskegee's role as a center of education for women in the years immediately before the Civil War. Later displays, interwoven with the end of Reconstruction and the beginning of the Jim Crow era, describe the creation of the Tuskegee Institute. One notes, "To retain power, white leaders looked for ways to appease new Negro voters. In Macon County, Negro voters wanted education." After briefly describing the political maneuvers to get funding for a school, the display notes, "The school and school's board of trustees . . . searched for and found an experienced, well-qualified young educator to start the new school. His name was Booker T. Washington." The display goes on to describe the partnership of the Tuskegee Institute with the philanthropist Julius Rosenwald, a trustee of the Institute and president of Sears Roebuck, to build schools for rural African Americans and to create an agricultural extension program that "became a model for USDA-sponsored cooperative extension services."

Finally, the displays in the first section highlight medical racism with the story of J. Marion Sims, the notorious father of gynecology who perfected his surgical techniques on female slaves.[41] The display text locates him within the borders of Macon County, observing that he "practiced medicine in the Cubahatchee community of Macon County from 1837–1840; developed many of his innovations while performing a series of experimental surgeries on a half dozen or so female slaves from Macon and surrounding counties between 1845 to 1849." It includes an even more substantial discussion of the slave Lucy Zimmerman, the first of the slaves Sims used in his experimental surgeries. A painting of Lucy on a table with Sims and two other white men standing over her is accompanied by text describing Zimmerman as "an unknown heroine of plantation society" who was the subject of medical experiments "a little more than one hundred years before the infamous Tuskegee Syphilis Study," and who was, like many of the men in the Study, forgotten by history.

The themes of multiculturalism, education, and medical racism are transformed by the movement across the last two sections of the center's exhibit. First, medical racism and abuse of research subjects—like Sims's experiments with female slaves and the Tuskegee Syphilis Study—are absent from the third section of the exhibit space. While all three areas address chronologically overlapping periods, only the first two areas discuss medical abuse and racism, thus reinforcing the positioning of the

lawsuit as the end of such practices. Additionally, the exhibit space devoted to the Study highlights how public awareness of the Study altered
the conduct of medical research. The display behind the lawsuit seal,
titled "In the Public Eye," details the Study becoming public in 1972
and the Clinton apology in 1997. The discussion of the Study becoming
public knowledge states:

> The public outcry over the Study was immense. Federal response to
> criticism of the Study, included HEW's formation of the Tuskegee
> Syphilis Study Ad Hoc Advisory Panel and inclusion of concerns about
> the study in the U.S. Senate hearings on human experimentation. Men
> in the Study—Herman Shaw, Charlie Pollard, Carter Howard, and
> Lester Scott—testified at the hearings. *Laws were passed that established pro-*
> *tocols on human experimentation and to protect the rights of participants.* In 1973 a
> lawsuit was filed by Fred Gray of the law firm of Gray, Seay & Lanford,
> on behalf of all the men in the Study. There was a government court
> approved settlement that included provisions for mandatory lifetime
> comprehensive medical care by the physician of their choice.[42]

Also, the bottom portion of the last panel, titled "The Legacy," observes,

> The Tuskegee Syphilis Study has medical, legal, social and physical
> legacies. Such legacies include its place in medical history as the lon-
> gest non-therapeutic experiment on human beings; the cause of new
> laws such as the National Research Act of 1974, which requires the
> establishment of Institutional Review Boards.

The center's spatial organization invites visitors to see the lawsuit over
the Study as the termination of medical abuses of African Americans,
and it discursively highlights legal outcomes, primarily the National
Research Act, as the way that research participants and patients are now
protected.

Second, the thematic foci of multiculturalism and education are
transformed into the legal pursuit for civil rights in the third part of the

exhibit space. As noted earlier, there are two freestanding, three-sided displays in the area. One is devoted entirely to issues involving the law and lawyers. The panel facing the open area of the second section is titled "Dixie Justice." It describes the importance of the law and the courts: "It was the law that guaranteed the right to vote, and on the most fundamental level, it was the law that set Negros free." This fact, the display indicates, was not lost on African Americans in the South:

> And, recognizing the importance of the laws in their fate, Negros struggled to gain admission to the legal profession despite doubts of capability, prejudice, and the risks that were often involved. Many of these lawyers were members of the National Bar Association. The quest for civil rights was a battle that took years, and is a battle that still endures. Without the parties willing to bring the suits, the lawyers willing to file the suits, and the judges willing to correctly interpret the law, the Civil Rights Movement would have been doomed.

The center emphasizes that the rights of African Americans depended on litigation. Visitors encounter a space that encourages affiliation with the center's thematic investment in a multiculturalism that becomes socially and rhetorically functional through litigation.

Yet, the litigation strategy faced a prior obstacle: legal education for African Americans. An inset box with the headline "The Negro Lawyer in Alabama" and a photograph of five African American lawyers during the Montgomery Bus Boycott makes this clear.[43] It begins:

> Entering the judicial system was no easy task for the first Negro lawyers in Alabama. There were no Negro universities that offered law degrees in the State of Alabama, and segregation prevented Negros from attending white law schools before the success of the Civil Rights Movement. . . . Negros who wanted to study law had to leave the state and return to Alabama upon graduation and pass the state bar examination. This presented additional difficulties for lawyers because refresher courses were not open to Negros (University of Alabama law graduates

did not have to take the state bar examination). Furthermore, once these lawyers finally began practicing in Alabama, they had to face the notorious discrimination and aggression that often met Negro lawyers, particularly those involved with civil rights.

The museum frames litigation as central to the civil rights struggle, while sidestepping the issue of local and state laws (and courts) that abetted discrimination. It also describes the challenges faced by aspiring African American lawyers to receive legal education, and makes the struggle for legal education the antecedent condition for the success of the civil rights movement.

The emphasis on legal education and litigation continues as you move around the freestanding display. The next section (located counterclockwise from "Dixie Justice") is titled "Righting Civil Wrongs" and is divided into two halves. The left half, "One Nation under Construction," describes the struggle for African American freedom and rights from the beginnings of slavery through the Civil War and the failure of Reconstruction. The bottom of this section is titled "Sowing the Seeds of Change: The Emergence of the Black Lawyer." Next to a picture of John Mercer Langston, founder of Howard University's School of Law, the display notes, "Colored people's entry into America's oppressive legal system occurred with the admission of Macon Bolling Allen in the Maine Bar in 1844. For the next seventy-five years, aspiring Colored attorneys struggled against the legal segregation, limited access to law schools and rejection from legal professional associations." It closes by describing the creation of the NAACP Legal Defense Fund, which in concert with the National Bar Association "was the foundation of the legal struggle for full citizenship and civil rights for blacks."[44] This narrative is reinforced by the organizational placement of African American lawyers as the culmination of the "construction" narrative that began with slavery, and it is also reinforced by the second half of the "Righting Civil Wrongs" display, which presents a timeline of national court cases and legislation devoted to civil rights, alongside a description of the National Bar Association as "America's legal conscience." This freestanding display brings the themes of education and multiculturalism from the first section of the museum to their apotheosis in the emphasis on legal education and the civil rights movement, especially its juridical and legislative successes. Organizationally, the material repeatedly positions references to lawyers and their importance either as the first, primary element in a display or as the final, culminating element. The text explicitly values lawyers and anthropomorphizes legal groups as the "foundation" for rights and the "conscience" of American law. Visitors are positioned as witnesses who affiliate in support of these lawyers.

The remainder of the section on civil rights provides additional details on the movement, including details about protests, marches, etc., but the placement and depiction of these events still reinforces the role of lawyers. The second freestanding display in the area discusses civil rights actions in Macon County and the role of Tuskegee Institute students. A section titled "Forgotten Marches and Protests" describes protests and marches through Tuskegee in solidarity with those harmed during Bloody Sunday in Selma. The text concludes with a description of legal action in relation to these events: "In the meantime, Tuskegee attorney Fred D. Gray and others were engaged in legal efforts to remove the injunction which held the marchers at bay in Selma." Along the back wall of this section, a timeline provides a broad history of the civil rights movement, with special emphasis on events in Macon County and in Alabama. Each color-coded section describes different protest actions that culminated in legal decisions supporting civil rights and ending segregation. At the bottom of each section is a set of drawers that present visitors with questions and interactive materials that emphasize the importance of education, voting, and service on juries. While broader than litigation, each of these interactive components frames the specific issue, whether school integration or voting, against the backdrop of the court cases that made school integration, voting, etc., possible. The timeline and exhibit space closes with the observation that the civil rights movement has had successes (e.g., the "crusade for citizenship was complete"), setbacks such as white flight from both urban centers and areas like Macon County, and the "challenges of governance" faced by African Americans who now controlled government in Tuskegee and Macon County.[45]

The Tuskegee History Center foregrounds memories of the Tuskegee Syphilis Study as an example of race and racism in America while also incorporating elements from the medical research narrative into its memory work. Visitors can also find brief references to the convoluted history of Booker T. Washington and the Tuskegee Institute that insinuate the memory of disgrace and shame into the warp and weft of the larger narrative. The first section of the museum discusses the beginning of Jim Crow. Booker T. Washington's Cotton States Exposition Address, or "The Atlanta Compromise" speech is featured prominently there. The exhibit includes one of eight audiovisual touchscreens found in the exhibit space.[46] The touchscreen allows visitors to listen to a recording of the speech, made by Washington in 1904 for Columbia records. The speech plays over a series of still images that begin with sharecroppers and their impoverished living conditions, and transitions to a portrait of Washington and images of the Tuskegee Institute community and its relatively better living conditions. The display text notes that Washington "recommended that freed slaves accept their socially inferior situation and focus instead on learning to support themselves economically" and that "many people, both Negro and white, interpreted his words as reinforcement for harsh Jim Crow laws of social repression against people of color."

Given the emphasis on civil rights throughout the center, such a depiction is damning, but it is moderated by later discussion of Washington in the section on civil rights. The timeline in the civil rights section opens with a discussion of the 1901 Alabama state constitution, which was designed to disenfranchise African Americans. The timeline entry for 1903 states, "Booker T. Washington discreetly gives financial support to legal battles for civil rights." That entry is associated with a drawer built into the base of the timeline containing additional information and interactive materials. One half of the drawer describes the issues that motivated the litigation, names the lawsuits that made it to the Supreme Court, and gives the outcomes. The other half describes "code words,"

like "His Nibs" and "The Wizard," used by Booker T. Washington's secretary and the lawyer arguing one of the cases against Alabama's 1901
constitution. The code words accompany the observation that

> Although Booker T. Washington did not publicly oppose the Alabama
> Constitution's clear disenfranchisement of blacks, he secretly financed
> and supported these legal cases. The fact that they made their way to
> the Supreme Court confirmed the need to continue financing lawsuits
> that tested the constitutionality of discriminatory laws.

The center as a whole paints a complex picture of Booker T. Washington,
as a man who publicly advocated the "separate but equal" doctrine while
at the same time financing the lawyers who would fight its most invidious
manifestations. Such depictions both support and complicate memories
that frame Washington's actions as a source of disgrace or shame.

The representation of Tuskegee Institute is similarly convoluted.
The first section of the exhibit space lauds the Institute's contributions
to education for African Americans, but in the section describing the
Study, the representation becomes more complicated. The description
of the Study—the part of the three-sided display in this area that faces
out toward the open exhibit space—downplays the role of the Institute
and Nurse Eunice Rivers, while the next section, moving counterclockwise around the display, gives it a larger role. One half of this display,
subtitled "Institutional Involvement," is crafted like an organizational
chart. At the very top is the United States Public Health Service, which
the chart notes "began, funded and recruited support for the full 40
years of the Study." After the PHS, the next tier of organizations is the
Alabama State Board of Health and the Tuskegee Institute's John A.
Andrew Hospital. Further down, the Tuskegee Institute is listed more
prominently than the National Institutes of Health. According to the
chart, "Tuskegee Institute was referred to as 'one of the leading examples
of Negro culture in this country,'" and "Dr. Robert R. Moton, principal
of Tuskegee Institute gave PHS permission to use the school's facilities." The arrangement of the chart and its discursive content operate in

tension with each other. The textual component recognizes that the PHS had the lead role while the Institute's part in the Study was minor, but the placement of Tuskegee in this organizational chart implies a greater complicity than the text describes.

Additionally, the last third of the display that describes the presidential apology for the Study condemns Tuskegee University and the Syphilis Study Legacy Committee:

> In February 1997, Atty. Fred Gray received a telephone call from a reporter asking when President Bill Clinton was going to be making an apology to the men of the Tuskegee Syphilis Study. Unknown to Atty. Gray, legal representative for the men, the Tuskegee Syphilis Legacy Committee [*sic*] had been established a year-and-a-half earlier, with one of its goals being to secure a presidential apology for the Study. In a parallel to the Study, the men who had not been informed of what was being done to their bodies during the Study, were again, not informed about efforts to secure a presidential apology for harm done to them, and for the government's involvement in the study.[47]

The display indicates that Gray and the men were not informed about the committee or its plans. It then compares the lack of information about the apology to the deceptions that surrounded the Study. Here, the relationship between the men of the Study and Tuskegee University is incorporated into memory narratives that imply the Institute and university deserve some measure of guilt and shame for their role in the Study and its aftermath.

The Tuskegee History Center crafts a memory of the Tuskegee Syphilis Study that situates visitors as witnesses to the legal successes against racist medical research. The lawsuit by the Study survivors is figured as pivotal to achieving civil rights in Macon County and in Alabama. As visitors walk through the center, they literally cross the lawsuit in order to leave a history of genocide, segregation, and medical abuse behind and enter a world shaped by African American lawyers and civil rights litigation, which brought the seeds of multiculturalism and educational attainment to fruition. This performance of memory foregrounds those public memories emphasizing race and racism, while incorporating memories of medical research throughout. Like other bioethical memories, it frames the National Research Act and the creation of IRBs and research oversight as the end of egregious medical research abuses like Tuskegee, but it moves beyond that by framing the legislation as part of a larger civil rights strategy of litigation and legislation. Like the lay memories of racism, it emphasizes the racist aspects of the Study and ties the Study to a broader history of medical abuse and racism, including the abuse of Lucy Zimmerman by J. Marion Sims. This medical racism, like segregation, is overcome through legal action. Finally, it presents a complicated picture of Booker T. Washington and Tuskegee University that resonates with memories emphasizing disgrace and shame while also complicating and troubling those memories. The center's presentation of this complicated history creates potential competition between its memories and those articulated at Tuskegee University's Legacy Museum.

THE LEGACY MUSEUM

Located on the campus of Tuskegee University, the Legacy Museum was first proposed in President Clinton's 1997 apology for the Study. In that speech, he promised the government would help Tuskegee University establish "a center for bioethics in research and healthcare," and that the center would "serve as a museum of the study and support efforts to address its legacy."[48] The Bioethics Center opened its doors in 2006, and the Legacy Museum was opened three years later.[49] The museum's website announces it was "created to honor the 599 participants of the United States Public Health Service Study of Untreated Syphilis in the Negro Male in Macon County, Alabama (1932–1972)."[50] Yet, despite these declarations of intent and the appearance of the new, PHS-centered name of the Study in two places, the Legacy Museum and the exhibits it contained in 2015 are characterized by a relative absence of material on the Study and the men enrolled in it, focusing instead on the Institute

and George Washington Carver's scientific and medical accomplishments.[51] Rhetorically, then, the museum is both an *ennoia* (an absence
or holding back of information, where the absence discloses or implies
what it hides) in regard to the Study, and a meditation on "legacy." Ennoia is one of several similar terms, including *paralipsis* and *circumlocutio,*
that speak to absences and lacunae in speech; but unlike those other
rhetorical figures, ennoia emphasizes absence without euphemism or
substituted language. The absence itself structures and discloses what
is not present. In contrast, a paralipsis occurs when the rhetor declares
they will not discuss a topic or issue that they name. The common example is some variation of "I will not talk about my opponent's drinking
and womanizing." Circumlocutio involves the use of a euphemism or
descriptive phrase in place of the name of the issue or object being addressed: The common example is to describe someone as "passing on"
who has died.

The Legacy Museum exists alongside a host of memorials to the accomplishments of Tuskegee Institute. Depending on how visitors exit
the interstate to drive into Tuskegee, they might pass the Tuskegee Airmen National Memorial and the Oaks, Booker T. Washington's home,
which is part of the Tuskegee Institute National Historic Site. As visitors
enter Tuskegee University on Booker T. Washington Blvd., they pass by
the George Washington Carver Museum (part of the Tuskegee Institute
National Historic Site) on their right, and a statue depicting Booker
T. Washington lifting the veil of ignorance from the slave on the left
(figure 2), which appeared in Ralph Ellison's *Invisible Man.* Next, one
passes the Tuskegee Cemetery, where Carver, Washington, and Robert
Moton (Tuskegee's second principal) are buried, along with many other
individuals whose names grace buildings and streets on campus. The
Legacy Museum and the National Bioethics Center are housed in the
former John A. Andrews Hospital's infantile paralysis center. Before one
even makes it to the museum, the university's contributions to education
and medicine for African Americans and scientific advances for all have
been affirmed multiple times. The campus wears its pride in its accomplishments on its sleeve. In light of that, discussing the Study could be

challenging, especially discussing those details that implicate members of the Institute's community, much less the Institute itself.

The museum takes up two floors in the former John A. Andrews Memorial Hospital's Infantile Paralysis wing. The Infantile Paralysis Unit was one of the few places dedicated to helping African American children with polio in the segregated South, but the hospital was also the location for the initial assessments of the men involved in the Study. Thus in this one space there exist points of pride and points of potential shame. Visitors are accompanied by a guide who explains the exhibits. The first-floor exhibit consists of art, primarily photographs by P. H. Polk, a photographer who spent the majority of his career in Tuskegee, where he documented life in the town and the Institute. The majority of the pictures feature George Washington Carver.[52] The second floor consists of two exhibits: the larger one is "The Patient, The Project, The Partnership: Mass Production & Distribution of HeLa Cells at Tuskegee University," and the other is "The United States Public Health Service Untreated Syphilis Study in the Negro Male, Macon County, Alabama, 1932–1972."

The museum's ennoia first requires changing the Study's name to distance it from the Institute/university. This task was primarily accomplished by the guides who said that the proper name for the Study was the "United States Public Health Service's Study of Untreated Syphilis in the Negro Male, Macon County, Alabama, 1932–1972" and *not* the "Tuskegee Syphilis Study."[53] Later, another guide speculated that the Tuskegee Institute had been deceived about the Study and "no one on campus really knew what had been happening."[54] The common name of the Study is disavowed, and casual comments about the Study further distance it from the Institute/university. The use of the new, longer name is justified by a small sign as one enters the exhibit dedicated to the Study. That sign, titled "Transforming the Legacy," reiterates the claims of the Syphilis Study Legacy Committee that the common name of the Study "obscures the achievements of Tuskegee (Institute) University in improving the health care of African Americans, indeed all Americans."

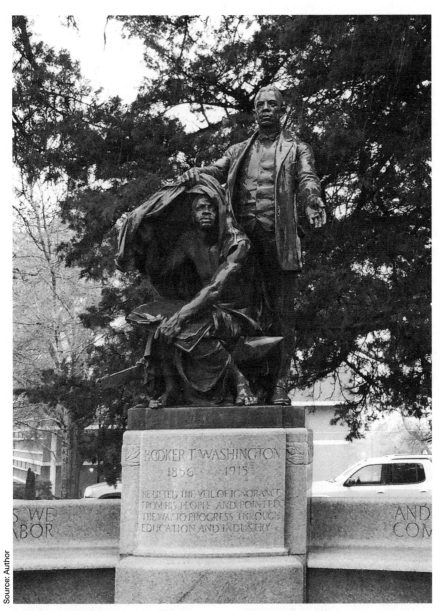

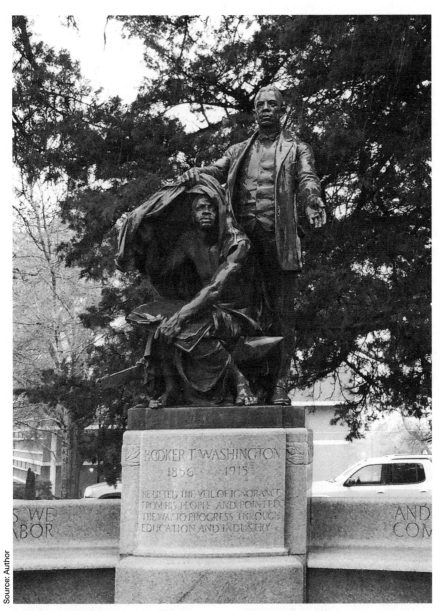

Figure 2. Statue of Booker T. Washington lifting the veil of ignorance from the face of the slave. This statue is found at the first intersection past the main gates of Tuskegee University. Visitors to campus must pass it to reach the Legacy Museum and the Tuskegee Institute National Historic Site. This statue is also referenced in Ralph Ellison's *Invisible Man*.

After this initial reference to the Study and an explanation of the museum's nomenclature for it, there are no details about the Study provided in the remainder of the exhibit. The displays focus on other ancillary issues. First, many displays focus on Clinton's apology for the Study. At the entrance to the exhibit, there is a photograph of six of the Study survivors, along with Bill Clinton, Al Gore, and surgeon general David Satcher on the day of the apology. Next is a framed picture of Bill Clinton greeting Myrtle Adams, who was a member of the Legacy Committee and chairwoman of the Macon County Health Care Authority, alongside the text of Clinton's apology. Visitors might also receive a one-page handout titled "Celebrating Fred Simmons." It includes a picture of Simmons, one of the survivors, and a series of bullet points detailing his life. The sheet, written by the museum staff, emphasizes details about Simmons or about the ceremony surrounding the apology, including observations about his age at the time of the apology (one hundred), his four generations of descendants, and how he refused to use a wheelchair while at the White House for the apology. Only two points about the Study itself are buried in the middle of the handout: The first, written in his voice, states, "I was an unwitting participant in this study from 1932–1972," and the second declares, "EVERYONE IN THE SYPHILIS STUDY WAS NOT POOR!" The details of this first display and the related handout emphasize a new name for the Study that dissociates it from Tuskegee, as well as celebrating the life of one survivor and the general importance of Clinton's apology to the survivors, the town, and the Institute.

The ennoiatic quality of the museum continues with the artifacts chosen for display. The exhibit includes a wide range of ancillary artifacts that reflect the broader cultural impact of the Study or discuss the prevalence and harms of syphilis without ever mentioning the Study explicitly. After seeing details of the apology, visitors are encouraged to move clockwise around the room. The next display is a 2003 Marvel Comics series, "Truth: Red, White & Black," that details a murderous eugenic program by the U.S. government that used black soldiers to create a "super soldier" serum, like that which produced Marvel's Captain

America. This is followed by 1930s-era PHS pamphlets about syphilis's dangers, two pictures displaying syphilitic sores on a woman's genitals, a playbill for *Miss Evers' Boys,* newspaper stories about the Clinton apology, a mimeograph of the HEW report on the Study, a series of drawings from a 1945 educational pamphlet titled "Corky the Killer," a display of the actual heavy metal treatments used to treat syphilis prior to 1946, a painting of sharecroppers produced by an artist who was debilitated by syphilis, and portraits of Eugene and Helen Dibble. With the exception of the heavy metal treatments, the exhibits are hung in a line at eye level around the room.

The contents of this exhibit are a hodgepodge of historical pamphlets, pop-culture reactions to medical racism, and reporting on the Clinton apology. Their visual interest is minimized by placing almost all the displays at eye level with no break in the exhibit's linearity. The only thematically coherent material—the material on Clinton's apology—is also the only material that breaks from the linear monotony of the displays. The arrangement of the displays works to minimize attention to the majority of the content. This also parallels the claims of one guide for how these materials are used. The guide claimed to use the materials on display as a springboard for discussion of contemporary racism and the ongoing danger of STDs like syphilis, especially for high school and college-aged visitors.

The exhibit on the Study is ennoiatic. The Study itself—details of those involved, what they did, who they did it to, etc., which were all present in the History Center—are absent from the Legacy Museum's exhibit on the Study. That absence can potentially disorient visitors. This occurs alongside the contrast between the laudatory view of the Clinton apology and the immediately subsequent presentation of the comic book series, with its murderous eugenic program. The exhibit space creates disorientation and confusion with its collection of objects: The disjointed presentation and the absence of the explicit unifying thread of the Study itself creates the space for the unheimlich to be experienced. This could lead to a positive ethical contemplation, where individuals reflect on the persistence of medical racism and racist beliefs about sexuality, implied by some of the exhibits, but it could also lead to a focus on a past that never was if objects like the Marvel comic book series become the focus of attention. The ambivalence of the unheimlich flowers in the absence fostered by ennoia.

The work of crafting a positive legacy for Tuskegee Institute, separate from the details of the Study, is performed in the other exhibits. As noted earlier, the first floor of the museum is dedicated to photographs of Tuskegee by a local artist. The photographs include images of Institute social events, family members of Institute and hospital leaders, the Tuskegee Airmen (including one photograph of a visit by Eleanor Roosevelt to Moton Airfield, where she flew with one of the Tuskegee Airmen), and multiple pictures of George Washington Carver. The pictures of Carver make up the entirety of one wall, and they include pictures of him working in a lab, painting, posing for a portrait, and talking with Henry Ford. Interspersed between the images are displays of equipment from Carver's laboratory, and in one corner, there is a poster from an academic conference, titled "Contributions of Dr. George Washington Carver to Global Food Security," describing innovations and discoveries by Carver that are still in use today.[55]

The photographs work to craft a positive legacy of Tuskegee. The images of Tuskegee emphasize the quality of life the Institute brought to the town. Others, like the picture of Eleanor Roosevelt, reinforce both the town's and the Institute's contributions to the larger civil rights movement and to the nation as a whole. The pictures from the Moton Airfield highlight the valuable contributions of Tuskegee and its eponymous airmen to the nation. According to the guides, the picture of Eleanor Roosevelt at the airfield was used by her to convince FDR to support the creation and deployment of the Tuskegee Airmen. The images of Carver reinforce his prominence as a scientist and a Renaissance man, which redounds to the Institute and its works as a whole. The discourse of the guides also reinforces what the images of Carver imply. For example, they indicated that the photograph of Carver and Henry Ford was taken *at Tuskegee:* Ford came to Carver, not the other way around. Similarly, the poster was used to emphasize not only scientific contributions but also philanthropy: neither Carver nor the Institute benefited financially from Carver's discoveries that have been employed to help so many others.

The Institute's contributions to biomedical advances for the sake of others is a central theme of the final exhibit in the museum. "The Patient, The Project, The Partnership" focuses on the Institute's role in distributing the HeLa cells used to culture the polio vaccine. The exhibit opens with the start of Tuskegee University's "First Bioethics Conference in Cancer Health Disparities Research in 2012." It was first used as a "trigger tool" to prompt discussion of the bioethical challenges raised by the derivation of the HeLa cells from Henrietta Lacks in 1951 without her consent or knowledge.[56] The exhibit opens with a floor-to-ceiling picture of Henrietta Lacks.[57] Here, the guides discussed how her dignity was discarded by doctors because she was a black woman, and they emphasized that such experiences of medical racism persist today. After the opening image of Lacks, visitors move counterclockwise around the room and encounter pictures of the men (Russell Williams and James H. M. Henderson) who ran the project at the Carver Foundation, and pictures of women working in the Carver Foundation laboratories to culture the HeLa cells and prepare them for shipment. The next display includes examples of correspondence between the Institute and other academic centers about the cells as well as the packing materials used to ship them. After description of the cell distribution, a timeline entitled "Henrietta, Everlasting" identifies the discoveries and inventions made possible by HeLa cells in various areas of biology.

After the timeline, the displays shift from the HeLa cell distribution project to discussing the present-day Comprehensive Cancer Center Partnership between the University of Alabama-Birmingham, Morehouse University, and Tuskegee University. This part of the exhibit includes two large academic poster presentations providing details about the partnership and Tuskegee's role in it, especially in the area of bioethics.[58] From there, the exhibit shifts to discussing the pre–Salk vaccine experience of childbirth and polio, especially the opening of the John A. Andrews maternity wing and the Infantile Paralysis Unit, where the museum is now housed. The wall displays close with several pictures of Dr. Salk and African American doctors, including an image of Salk and the doctors immunizing African American babies with the Salk vaccine. There are also a variety of freestanding displays that exhibit items from the Carver Foundation, such as a typewriter, microscope, and other lab paraphernalia, and items from the Infantile Paralysis Unit, including leg braces and wheelchairs for polio sufferers that had been crafted by Tuskegee Institute students.

This exhibit prompts public feelings of affiliation and the unheimlich through its meditation on African American contributions to medical research. Visitors witness in the displays both the accomplishments of Tuskegee and the medical racism the Institute and all African Americans faced. The exhibit depicts Tuskegee as a contributor to past research on cell biology and vaccine testing and a contributor to contemporary re-search on cancer. It also shows how African Americans like Henrietta Lacks have been treated as a source of material for biological research, with no knowledge or opportunity to agree to participate. Tuskegee University is situated as trying to contribute to medical science and im-prove the lives of African Americans while societal and medical racism permitted the violation of black bodies.

This exhibit also highlighted, if unwittingly, the dependence of the Tuskegee Institute on the largesse of the federal government, especially the PHS. Guides noted that Tuskegee Institute/University did not profit from its work in the HeLa cell project. Government funding instead went into paying for laboratory upkeep and was used to provide training opportunities for Tuskegee Institute students. Yet the discussion stops with the existence of that dependence rather than a consideration of how such dependence on the government might inform our understanding of the Syphilis Study and the (in)capacity of the Institute to stop it. Even as the HeLa exhibit and the Carver materials meditate on the posi-tive medical contributions, the ennoia rendering the negative medical impact of the Syphilis Study structures and limits the types of witness-ing and contemplation of medical racism that are possible.

Memory and Agon

The public revelation of the "Tuskegee Syphilis Study" produced a rich memory culture that exemplifies the multiple, partial, and conflicting qualities of memory. The memory practices embodied in bioethical and public texts have offered visions of the Study as the justification for re-search regulation, especially around the issue of informed consent, and as an exemplar of American racism in medicine. Yet for some, especially those affiliated with Tuskegee University, the memories of the Study also provoke shame and a desire to rename the Study to emphasize the role of the PHS and diminish any link to the city or the university. The two museums reflect this extant memory culture, but even as they reflect it, they also select and deflect attention from various aspects of that memory culture.

The Tuskegee History Center's account of the Study blends the memories of race and racism and memories of medical research: Visitors witness a memory narrative that frames the Study as a result of racism and brutality. It resolves that story of racism in medicine and public life by centering—symbolically and physically—the lawsuit filed by survivors as the moment when the region and the country shifted from a history of racism into a timeless present of civil rights achieved through litigation and the courts. The center offers a rich historical narrative detailing the actions of African, European, and Native Americans in Alabama, and it centers Macon County and Alabama as the epicenter of civil rights activity. This is altogether fitting considering that Macon County is the birthplace of Rosa Parks and Fred Gray, and that Alabama was a hotbed for civil rights agitation and protest. The center also invokes the local memories of disgrace and shame, but those memories are presented in an ambivalent fashion. The center recalls that Washington quietly sup-ported civil rights legislation but also advocated for a "separate but equal" view of European and African Americans. It describes the role Tuskegee Institute played in the Syphilis Study. It emphasizes how the university excluded Fred Gray and the surviving men in the Study from the campaign for a presidential apology and ignores the history of the lawsuit that forced the university and the CDC to exclude Gray and the men from the initial planning. Yet the center notes that the PHS led the Study and describes the lawsuit as focused solely on the federal government and white doctors, reflecting Gray's view during the lawsuit in the 1970s that the Institute was not legally culpable for the Study.

The center's performance of memory positions visitors as witnesses who affiliate (or feel *philia*) in celebrating these civil rights accomplishments and recognizing themselves (and the broader nation) as a people of laws and civil rights. Yet the center's performance of memory, which culminates in a timeless civil rights moment, cannot account for the need for ongoing struggle against racism in both medicine and society at large, even as the center's final display closes with the recognition that civil rights struggles must continue. Its focus on litigation is understandable given that a successful civil rights lawyer spearheaded its creation, but that focus is troubling because all other protest strategies that constituted the civil rights movement are subordinated to litigation. This is not to critique litigation or imply that Gray is wrong for wanting to remember the successes to which he contributed. Rather, the overweening focus on litigation obscures the broader social activism that shifts racist attitudes and cultural standards so that subsequent legislation can succeed. It also fails to consider what the ascendancy of a conservative judiciary means for future litigation in the name of civil rights and social justice, and the risk that such an ascendant conservatism poses to the movement's accomplishments.

The Legacy Museum offers a complex rhetorical mediation of those memory cultures framed around an ennoia, an absence that traces the outline of what is missing. Details of the Study and much of the racism in the region are absent, but it is an absence that ironically calls attention to itself. This can be seen most clearly in the fact that the Study itself is not discussed, but Clinton's apology for the undescribed Study is. Instead, the museum explicitly considers multiple "legacies" of the Tuskegee Institute: The museum describes how the Institute/university has a legacy of struggling against racism and working to improve the lives of African Americans through education and medicine. This is made most prominent in its depiction of George Washington Carver and the Institute's role in distributing HeLa cells for producing the polio vaccine. The museum does honor the survivors of the Study, primarily through its supplemental material about Fred Simmons, but its very act of honoring also deflects attention away from the very reason their survival deserves commemoration. The museum's ennoia can foster feelings of the unheimlich in visitors who contemplate medical racism amidst details of the Tuskegee Institute's legacy, but this assumes that visitors are familiar enough with the Study to fill in the museum's absence. Those lacking that knowledge will have an experience grounded solely in the discourses on legacy.

The museum's ennoia is driven at least in part by memories of the Study as something shameful abetted by the university. These memories also highlight the broader struggle of memory regarding the place of Booker T. Washington and the Institute in recollections of civil rights activism, and the classism that marked Washington's work. These memories often take the form of hints and insinuations that are made powerful by their implication and absence. That absence also makes it difficult to challenge them explicitly. The museum therefore responds while sidestepping the challenges of directly addressing those insinuations. The museum is placed within the university's memory culture—recalling Washington, Carver, positive work that occurred contemporaneously with the Study, and tying that to the university's present actions and accomplishments—all while leaving the Study itself absent. The possibility of defamation has shaped the Legacy Museum, the temporalities and gaps in the "legacy" it offers, and its abjuration of the Study and its commonplace name, even as the memory of the "Tuskegee Syphilis Study" leads some to visit.

None of this is to lay blame for the Study at the feet of the Tuskegee Institute or to detract from its hard work in the past and in the present to improve the lives of African Americans across the nation and in Macon County. As others have noted, the PHS was solely responsible for designing the Study and keeping it active for more than forty years. Yet, focusing solely on that fact and obscuring the details of the Study hide the complicated history of the Institute—and all African American institutions—in the Jim Crow South, where the survival of the institutions and the communities they represented involved a complicated balance between avoiding the violence of their segregationist white neighbors, appealing to Northern white philanthropists and the federal government, and aiding their communities to the best of their abilities.[59] In such an environment, failure is inevitable: Not all interests can be appeased, especially when one of the parties (i.e., Southern whites) was invested in degrading their black neighbors. As Manning Marable and others have noted, these conditions encouraged classism—distinguishing and protecting the black middle class in comparison to others like the poorer sharecropping communities in Macon County. Such a quality is reinforced by the Legacy Museum handout declaring not all men in the Study were poor. That classism might have made it easier for some members of the Tuskegee Institute community, like Robert Moton, Eugene Dibble, and others identified by James Jones, to agree to facilitate the PHS's Study in Macon County.

Both the Tuskegee History Center and the Legacy Museum embody the public memory and bioethical memory of the Tuskegee Syphilis Study, but they subordinate the memory of research to the public memory of race and racism so that, while consequential, the memory of research is now situated as another harm inflicted on African Americans as a whole, rather than a uniquely evil event in medicine. While they are united in how they situate the bioethical and public memories of the Study, they also exist in tension with each other. The center at different moments condemns the university that houses the museum, and by placing litigation and lawyers at the pinnacle of the civil rights movement, it does not consider the ways that racism's micropolitics are beyond the law's purview. The marked absence of the Study from the museum obfuscates the reason some individuals visit it, as well as the federal impetus for its creation. Additionally, if members of the public have visited the center and seen its history of Washington's acquiescence to post-Reconstruction segregation and the Tuskegee Institute's role in the Study, the museum's exhibits are mute on this issue and depend on the guide's rhetorical finesse to address this. Given the overwhelming commitment to absence and ennoia, this will render such discussions problematic, both because visitors might lack the information to consider these issues and because any discussion of the Study could be interpreted as an attack on the Tuskegee Institute's legacy.

But if both sites are visited, the combined visit can provide a "memorial agon," where tension and conflict between specific partial memories lead to richer, more nuanced experiences and understandings of memory and history by visitors.[60] Here, a memorial agon operates in the gaps between the presented materials at both sites and the differing temporal orientations of each site's material. The History Center makes present details of the Study and the successes of the civil rights movement even as its timeless present renders an understanding of the civil rights movement *as ongoing, incomplete, and awaiting a future apotheosis* somewhat difficult to grasp. The Legacy Museum renders the Study absent, even as that absence calls attention to itself. It further emphasizes the ongoing struggles against racism in medicine and in the broader culture, a topic that guides are trained to emphasize and discuss with visitors. Temporally, the center takes us through the past, including the "past" of the Study, into a present marked by the civil rights movement. The museum looks forward to the struggles against racism that must continue. The tensions between the two can be resolved by viewing each as offering a temporal orientation left unconsidered by the other. Visitors themselves encounter both and thus have the agency to witness and to resolve the agon and tension between the two sites. Visitors encounter the tension in the two museums' positions alongside their complementary content, allowing for a contemplation of both the struggles of the past found at the History Center and the challenges for a better, nonracist future indicated by the Legacy Museum. Similar dynamics, unfortunately, are not found in public memorializing about other events in bioethics's origin story.

CHAPTER 4

Minimal Remembrance and the Obligation to Remember

OFFICIAL AND VERNACULAR MEMORIES OF THE WILLOWBROOK STATE SCHOOL

———•◆•———

On January 6, 1972, viewers of New York City's ABC affiliate were introduced to the horrible conditions at the Willowbrook State School, a state institution for the developmentally disabled. With the help of one of the doctors, a young Geraldo Rivera and a two-man camera crew made an unannounced visit to one of the school's wards. Over images of children—some naked, some covered in filth, all neglected—a shaken Rivera observed,

> The doctor had warned me it would be bad. It was horrible. There was one attendant for perhaps 50 severely and profoundly retarded children. Children lying on the floor naked and smeared with their own feces. They were making a kind of pitiful sound, a kind of mournful wail that it is impossible for me to forget.
>
> This is what it looked like. This is what it sounded like, but how

can I tell you about the way it smelled? It smelled of filth; it smelled of disease; and it smelled of death.[1]

That evening and the next day, ABC received over seven hundred telephone calls expressing outrage at the conditions at Willowbrook.[2] Other journalists immediately visited to file their own stories.

Yet, this was not the first time scandal had surrounded Willowbrook. Since its opening in 1951, the institution had been overcrowded, understaffed, and a breeding ground for measles, shigella, and hepatitis. These conditions had been repeatedly covered in local papers. The institution received state and national attention in the mid-sixties when Robert Kennedy made a surprise visit and declared after touring one of the wards that Willowbrook was "a snakepit."[3] Yet, unlike the previous scandals that had failed to spark change, Rivera's exposé led to a 1975 lawsuit and a consent judgment where the State of New York agreed to phase out Willowbrook and other large institutions for the developmentally disabled under the oversight of the Willowbrook Review Panel; but this would be a contentious process that would take more than twelve years to complete.[4] Embedded in this story of institutional horror and neglect is a story of dubious medical research. Infectious diseases spread rapidly through the Willowbrook School's population, as they did in other institutions for the developmentally disabled. The school worked with New York University's Saul Krugman to study the transmission of hepatitis. The goal was to eliminate or curtail the spread of the disease. Krugman and his research team began a series of studies that ran from 1954 to 1972, but the experiments raised profound ethical questions.[5] Today, Willowbrook appears alongside Tuskegee in bioethics training as unethical research that violates tenets of autonomy, beneficence, and justice.[6]

The story of Krugman and his research is part of the larger story of Willowbrook, a story with a great deal of affective power. The raw horror at Willowbrook's conditions and attempts to respond to that in public memory swamp public recollection of Krugman's experiments. On the one hand, Willowbrook's conditions should be foregrounded for historical and ethical reasons: Epidemic hepatitis could only exist because of the squalor at Willowbrook, which was enabled by collective neglect. That neglect and the diseases that followed enabled Krugman's research. Yet, it is notable that public memory rarely calls Krugman's research to mind. Only one artifact that I have found discusses it. We can make sense of this by staying a moment with the horror of Willowbrook. That horror demanded and continues to demand a response from state actors and the broader public called to act as witnesses. Yet in addition to demanding our witness, the horror and disgust and outrage provoked by images from Willowbrook also harms the reputation of state actors who allowed these conditions to persist and, as this chapter will explain, fought the closure of the school. Public memory is "animated by affect,"[7] but that animation can drive the producers of public memory toward acts of *minimal remembrance* just as easily as it could encourage them to engage in thoughtful witnessing. However, not all creators of public memory are stained by the horrors of Willowbrook equally.

To make sense of the different responses to Willowbrook and Krugman's experiments, we can turn to an older distinction in public memory research: official public memory and vernacular public memory. Official public memory of the school offers a "minimal remembrance" of Willowbrook. This memory work forecloses recollection of the school by taking the rhetorical form of a "monument" that fashions heroic actors who vanquished the horror of Willowbrook and closed the school. Vernacular public memory does not have the need for minimal remembrance, and in contrast with official memory, it highlights the horrible conditions at the school and the neglect that enabled it in order to reinforce public commitment to supporting care for the developmentally disabled. Finally, the one vernacular memory piece that addresses Krugman's research must literally sanitize both the school and the experiment in order to allow audiences to act as witnesses to problematic medical research.

A Brief History of Willowbrook and Krugman's Research

Americans began building state-supported large institutions for the developmentally disabled in the second half of the nineteenth century, although state support for building these institutions waxed and waned from one decade to the next.[8] Willowbrook was built during a period of remarkable growth for state institutions. According to James W. Trent, "Between 1950 and 1970, state authorities built, refurbished, and added to more public facilities than any other period of their history."[9] Yet, even as institutions grew, their populations exploded, growing twice as fast as the general population from 1946 to 1967.[10] Willowbrook State School opened in April 1951. From the beginning, the school faced challenges. Of all New York institutions, Willowbrook housed more of the most profoundly disabled individuals in the New York system, which was a problem for Willowbrook since institutions depended on less disabled individuals housed there to work at the institution in order for it to remain financially viable.[11] By 1969, over three-quarters of Willowbrook's residents were classified as "profoundly or severely retarded."[12] From the outset, the school was overcrowded: in 1955, about 3,600 people occupied facilities designed for 2,950.[13] Local newspapers reported incidents of violence, abuse, and death in the school as early as 1952.[14] States were building new institutions for the developmentally disabled, but they were not maintaining or adequately staffing them, thus encouraging squalor.

And squalor bred disease. Of specific concern was hepatitis, which was believed to be widespread or even endemic to the school (i.e., it was believed all residents and staff were infected).[15] At the time, the transmission of the disease and its progress was poorly understood, so Saul Krugman began a series of experiments to better understand the transmission and prevention of the disease.[16] The first experiment assessed how many Willowbrook residents had hepatitis and whether injections of gamma globulin, the component of human blood rich in antibodies, would protect individuals from infection.[17] While some protective effect was shown, the results raised additional questions for Krugman and his colleagues. This led to a second set of experiments during which Krugman opened a separate unit in Willowbrook with its own admission protocols. The unit was separate from the larger school and required explicit parental consent to enroll children in the ward and the study. Here, Krugman's team fed live virus to children by feeding them chocolate milk laced with hepatitis-infected feces.[18] They then injected some children with the protective gamma globulin but not others, and then fed all of them the virus-laced feces mixture again. This study incidentally led to the observation that some children would suffer a second attack of hepatitis several months after the initial infection, which led Krugman to hypothesize that two different viruses were at work. To assess this hypothesis, he started a third round of experiments in which his team would admit groups of children to the special unit in the school and feed them virus from the pooled collection of all viruses at Willowbrook or specifically isolated samples thought to contain different viruses. The timing of those different exposures and the subsequent courses of disease in these children supported Krugman's hypothesis that two different viruses were at work—viruses we know today as Hepatitis A and Hepatitis B.

While many laypeople react with horror to Krugman's studies, he had vociferous defenders within medicine. Krugman received multiple awards from medical societies for his hepatitis research, including the Markle Foundation's John Russell award for his "impact and influence on medicine" and a Lasker Award for Public Service in 1983, the highest award for research in the United States.[19] Allen Weise describes Krugman as one of the men who provided "the keys to unlocking the solution" to hepatitis.[20] This does not mean that Krugman's work was ignored by medical researchers and ethicists. The ethical problems in Krugman's Willowbrook experiments were first brought to light by Henry K. Beecher in 1966. Beecher included Krugman's experiments in his list of twenty-two cases of unethical research published in the *New England Journal of Medicine*.[21] Krugman's research received additional attention when members of the Progressive Labor Party (PLP) and the Medical Committee for Human Rights (MCHR) protested his continuing research and the recognition it received from the American College of Physicians in 1972.[22] The protests about Krugman's research may have led to a symposium held at New York University's School of Medicine, where Krugman, bioethicists, and his critics discussed the study.[23]

Critics of Krugman's research identified four issues with his study. At the symposium, critics derided his study for deliberately infecting children with hepatitis, conducting research that has no direct benefit for the children who participate, coercing consent (i.e., admission to Krugman's unit was open when the school itself was closed to new admissions, thus forcing parents to enroll in the study if they wanted help for their severely disabled children), and for using the horrific conditions at Willowbrook to justify experimenting on the children.[24] These points are amplified in the criticism by David and Sheila Rothman. In their book on Willowbrook, they observe, "If Willowbrook was hell for its residents, it could be paradise for a researcher. On these disease-ridden wards, the line between treatment and experimentation seemed to vanish."[25] They argue that this blurred line is found in the consent form Krugman had parents sign, which "encourages parents to commit their children to the unit" and claims "the team is 'studying' hepatitis, not doing research" and describes "introducing the live virus as 'a new form of prevention,' but feeding a child hepatitis hardly amounted to prevention."[26] Furthermore, they argue that Krugman does not deserve plaudits for helping cure hepatitis; that recognition, they argue, belongs solely to Dr. Baruch Blumberg, who "was actually solving the problem in his laboratory, without conducting experiments on humans."[27]

These arguments, especially those by the Rothmans, did not go unanswered. In fact, the most ardent defender of Saul Krugman was Saul Krugman, who participated in the NYU symposium, was the object of a fawning 1974 interview in *Modern Medicine,* and published an extensive defense of his work in 1986.[28] Ultimately, though, the concerns raised by Beecher and others carried the day and became incorporated into the memory practices of bioethics. Willowbrook joined Tuskegee as an exemplar of research run amok, but those bioethical memories, while prominent for medical research, are overshadowed in the public sphere by official acts of minimal remembrance and vernacular condemnation of the institution as a whole.

Minimal Remembrance and Monumental Form

Official public memory often works to stabilize and circulate self-aggrandizing identities of nations and institutions. Such work must manage the often uncomfortable histories of our institutions. I argue here that Willowbrook's official public memory operates as a minimal remembrance facilitated by a distinctly monumental form for the composition of memory. Monuments are functionally different from memorials, although both are material enactments of public memory. According to Marita Sturken, "Monuments are not generally built to commemorate defeats; the defeated dead are remembered in memorials. Whereas a monument most often signifies victory, a memorial refers to the life or lives sacrificed for a particular set of values."[29] Monumental history and memory focus on heroes or heroic accomplishments; the public memories instantiated in monumental form offer a celebratory vision of the past that requires little detail or explanation beyond the basic recognition of the hero. The fact that the accomplishment exists is sufficient; no exploration of causes or context is required. As Nietzsche argues in his description of monumental forms of history, the harm imposed by monumental history and memory is that "the past itself suffers *damage:* very great portions of the past are forgotten and despised, and flow away like a grey uninterrupted flood, and only single embellished facts stand out as islands."[30]

One outcome of monumental forms then is that they operate rhetorically to deflect attention away from unflattering aspects of the past. They focus the visitor's attention on elements of memory that can be displayed epideictically, and, if possible, in mythic terms. Monumental forms of memory disentangle history and memory, severing ties between the two, in the name of triumphal recollection.[31] According to Sturken, an exemplar of this form of public memory can be found in the Washington Monument: Beyond its name, there is little in that white marble obelisk to remember the man or his achievements. No image of Washington graces the monument bearing his name; no words of his appear on its surface. All that remains are the pure phallic geometry of the object and a denotative connection to the United States' first president.

This rhetorical effect can be drawn into sharper relief when compared to the rhetorical form of memorials, which focus on those who have suffered or died for a cause. In their remembrance of the dead, memorials are often pedagogical, providing details about the historical past as well as the moral lessons that one should draw from it. Sturken identifies the Lincoln Memorial and the Vietnam Veterans Memorial as exemplars here: both remember the dead through explicit naming on the memorial, and, in the case of the Lincoln Memorial, the values visitors should learn are made explicit through the inscription of Lincoln's words on the memorial's walls.

In this way, *the rhetorical form of the monument encourages minimal remembrance,* a recognition that a past event happened, while forgetting the causes and conditions that led to the event being remembered. What is recalled by the monument is the bare minimum required to sustain a denotative connection and foster epideictic recall. Complications and nuance that impede the monument's celebratory mode are set aside. Yet, while these monuments try to maintain their rhetorical purity, no site or artifact of public memory is pure in its form or content. All are contaminated by the places and discourses that surround them. The Washington Monument, for example, is surrounded by ancillary rhetorics that describe and emplace it, even as the main monument downplays or effaces the contents of memory. In its primary function of effacing the past, then, monumental form and minimal remembrance are an ideal mode for official memory that seeks to contain traumatic events and images, like those that surround Willowbrook.

OFFICIAL MEMORY WORK AT THE CSI/WILLOWBROOK SITE

Official memory work began with the official closing of the Willowbrook School in 1987. Woven through the official memory work is a desire to deflect attention from the state's role in Willowbrook's squalor. On the former Willowbrook site, now the College of Staten Island (CSI), are two permanent memorials to the school. The first is a commemorative plaque, emplaced at the official close of the school on September 17, 1987

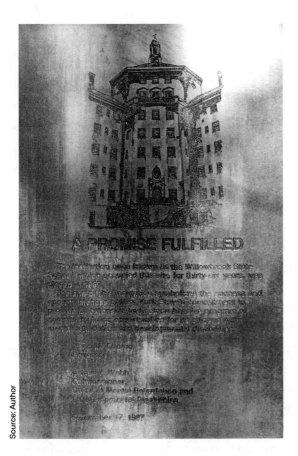

Source: Author

Figure 3. Willowbrook commemorative plaque. The plaque was placed in 1987 and is located at the center of the College of Staten Island's campus. Until 2013, the plaque was not accessible to those with mobility issues.

(figure 3). Located in a small grove of trees at the center of CSI's campus, the plaque is engraved with an image of Building 2, which had been the main building at the Willowbrook School.[32] Under the headline "A Promise Fulfilled," the following statement appears:

> The institution once known as the Willowbrook State School, which occupied this site for thirty-six years, was closed in 1987.
>
> The end of this institution symbolizes the success and appropriateness of New York State's commitment to provide an extensive and comprehensive program of community living opportunities for its citizens with mental retardation and developmental disabilities.

It closes with the names of the governor and commissioner of the Office of Mental Retardation and Developmental Disability (OMRDD), respectively, at the time of the closure: Mario Cuomo and Arthur Webb. This plaque is affixed to a large rock located in a small grove of trees. For most of the memorial's existence, there was no sidewalk or access for people with physical disabilities. In late 2013, apparently in response to the publication of David Goode and colleague's *A History and Sociology of the Willowbrook State School,* which observed that the monument was not accessible to those with disabilities,[33] CSI installed a paved path, ending in an open area with a bench and some landscaping (figure 4).

The other memory site on campus is the Building 19 monument. Willowbrook's buildings were numbered, not named.[34] They were all marked at the entrances and corners of the buildings with black numbers in a white circle. After Willowbrook closed, many buildings were refurbished for use in the new educational setting of the College of Staten Island. Part of the renovation involved changing the layout of the building. Original entrances were removed, and they become architectural follies, often holding the window for an office or central hallway. The back doors of the buildings were made the main entrance, and if the building had two stories, the old fire escapes were replaced with an enclosed stairwell. The building numbers were sandblasted off all the CSI buildings, except for one. During my visit, I was told that as the college moved into the Willowbrook property, some faculty objected that the changes to the buildings were intended to "erase" Willowbrook. The memorial on Building 19, now CSI's school of education, is the official response to that protest, and the sole attempt to maintain some element of the old buildings. On the back corner of the building, facing a path leading from the green space surrounding the library to a faculty/staff parking lot, one can find a sun-faded "19" in a white circle and a small plaque (figure 5). In front of the plaque and number, a rose bush has been planted. The plaque reads, "To honor those who struggled on the grounds of the Willowbrook Institution we preserve this former building number in their respected remembrance."

The events remembered at Willowbrook clearly are not as memorable

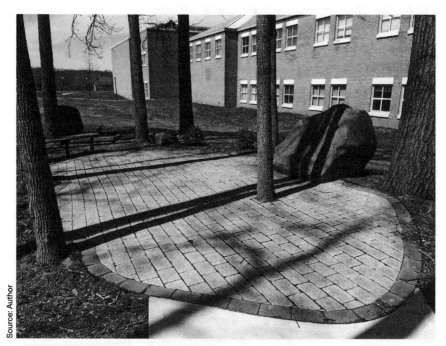

Source: Author

Figure 4. Willowbrook commemorative plaque and paved area. The plaque was installed on the former school grounds in 1987, but the paved area that makes it accessible to those with mobility issues was installed in 2013.

as the "father of the country." Therefore, the complete discursive absence and geometric abstraction of the Washington Monument is impossible to achieve. Nonetheless the monuments perform a monumental form of memory that has three specific effects. First, the explicit content of these two monuments position some individual or group as the hero. The 1987 plaque praises the state for closing Willowbrook and turning to community housing models of care for those with developmental disabilities. The plaque frames those actions as a "success" of the state. On one hand, this is accurate: New York did close Willowbrook and did shift to community housing models of care. Yet, the remembrance shaped here forgets that New York ran Willowbrook in the first place and was forced to close the school by legal action. It also sidesteps the fact that the state fought the implementation of the court's decree at

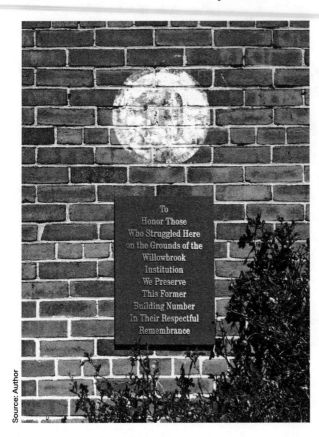

Figure 5. Building 19 Memorial is located on the corner of the building housing CSI's education school. A rose bush was planted in front of the number and plaque.

every possible step.[35] While the 1987 memory work glorifies the state, the Building 19 memorial offers praise to an ambiguous group. It glorifies "those who struggled" at Willowbrook, language that is reminiscent of the civil rights movement and its "struggles," while deflecting attention from the fact that whoever "they" were, they were struggling against the state.

Second, both of these monuments obscure the abject conditions of Willowbrook's residents. In the 1987 plaque, closing Willowbrook is framed as a good, but why that closure is a good thing is ambiguous, unless individuals recall the horrible conditions at the school. While individuals who attended the ceremony officially closing the school were likely familiar with its history, it is not clear that others in 1987 or since then would recall the conditions at the school. Similar work happens with the Building 19 monument's praise of "those who struggled" at the school. This language overlooks the fact that residents of Willowbrook were some of the most profoundly disabled individuals in the state's care, and the majority (but not all)[36] of them were incapable of struggle in the civil rights movement sense of struggle implied here. The Building 19 memorial praises a group of "those who struggled" that did not exist. When combined with the glorification of New York State in the 1987 plaque, the extant monuments on the former Willowbrook site deflect attention from the abject condition of many of its residents.

Third, both monuments and the work that made them possible foreclose the middle voice that facilitates memory and erases material traces of Willowbrook. The monuments' rhetorical structure creates emotional and narrative closure that precludes the middle voice of much public memory work. The middle voice of public memory emphasizes the relationship between an object, image, or artifact of public memory and the viewer or spectator: It involves "state of mind, attitude, temporal and sequential positioning . . . [and] those aspects of the image that help the spectator develop that relationship."[37] Both monuments use active voice and past tense—the state's closure of the school "symbolizes" its commitment, while the college actively "preserves" the Building 19 signage to "honor" people. The use of past tense provides narrative and emotional closure. The events exist firmly in the past, and the monument works to remind us that the event *happened* but not that it has continued meaning or salience for people today. The past recalled by the monuments has been closed off and superseded by new approaches to caring for those with developmental disabilities.

Alongside the work performed by the content of the monuments, the construction of the monuments and the repurposing of the Willowbrook site works to substantially forget the conditions that existed at the school. When the campus was renovated, the architectural components most emblematic of the school were destroyed. Many buildings were demolished, specifically Building 2, which was the iconic building associated with the school and which housed Saul Krugman's hepatitis experiments. One of the most potent symbols of the school—and the building freighted with some of the most disturbing history (for bio-ethics, at least)—was destroyed. In addition to the demolition of some buildings, the renovation of the remainder reoriented the buildings and how visitors interact with them. The original entrances were eliminated, metal grates covering the windows were removed, and the old number-ing system was mostly eliminated. In many ways, this physical reshap-ing of the place undermines the material substrate that enables the creation and circulation of public memory. The relationships between viewers and the objects of potential memory were foreclosed symboli-cally, and the material objects that would cue memory were themselves eliminated.

These three qualities of the official memory work at the CSI/ Willowbrook campus—valorizing the state, obscuring conditions at Willowbrook, and eliminating physical traces that could prompt memory—create a monumental form of memory that fosters minimal remembrance. Official memory work contains Willowbrook's history by valorizing New York State and producing a sense of historical closure. It eliminates material traces that could prompt other memories, and it also articulates Willowbrook as part of a different and archaic era, implying that the shameful conditions at Willowbrook cannot be repeated. To the extent that this work fosters bioethical memory, it calls individuals together as witnesses to the heroic work of the state. This deflects atten-tion from the struggle to improve the lives of those at Willowbrook and the hard work by non-state actors to realize that improvement.

Likely, much of this minimal remembrance is not accepted by visi-tors to these monuments, especially if they recall the fact that the state ran Willowbrook. State and college officials were likely aware of this, as it was not until two years ago that the plaque was easily accessible: There was no paved access to the plaque, even though the plaque was located near the center of campus. Equally problematic is the possibility that the monumental form's closure of the past could be successful, even as its valorization of the state is not. The sense that care has improved and history has been overcome comports with common progressive views of history. Minimally remembering Willowbrook, then, is to remember a dead past that cannot haunt us, rather than recalling a past that demands our witness and a response to its injustices.

Monumental form also operates in official memory work that circulated outside of the former Willowbrook campus. In 2012, on the anniversary of Geraldo Rivera's exposé, the Office for Persons with Developmental Disabilities (OPWDD) opened its traveling exhibit "Remembering Willowbrook" at the New York Port Authority. The exhibit traveled the state for the next year. It now resides at the CSI archives. The exhibit offers substantially more detail about Willowbrook and the conditions at the school. It also continues the monumental forms' creation of heroes, although here the role of hero is shared between the state and Geraldo Rivera.

Each location would add different additional materials to the exhibit, but all iterations of the exhibit included a rocking horse from one of the child units at Willowbrook, a wheelchair that had been commonly used in all of Willowbrook's wards and buildings, and a series of pasteboard displays offering a timeline of the Willowbrook School's history and the work of OPWDD after Willowbrook was closed, which is the main component of the exhibit.[38] The timeline includes ten display boards. With the exception of the introductory board, a timeline runs through the middle of each display, surrounded by photographs and newspaper clippings detailing events at specific points on the timeline. The introductory board presents the exhibit's name under the seal of the OPWDD. Under that is a series of three pictures: one showing a Halloween parade on Willowbrook's grounds, one showing the demolition of a Willowbrook building, and one showing the decay of a former Willowbrook building that is unoccupied by CSI or OPWDD.[39] The introductory text below the pictures notes the official closing of the school in 1987: "Governor Mario Cuomo stated that the former Willowbrook School was officially and forever closed." The language of "officially and forever" reinforces the heroic framing of official public memory at CSI and its placement of Willowbrook's horror firmly in the past.

The introductory board then begins the heroic framing of Rivera, with the observation that the official closure of Willowbrook "came on the 15th anniversary of Geraldo Rivera's exposé." According to the text, Rivera's exposé built on a slow groundswell of outrage about the treatment of individuals with developmental disabilities, and "it was from the stories of neglect, abuse, and more, as well as the inspiring dedication and advocacy of parents and loved ones, that a state agency dedicated to serving people with intellectual and developmental disabilities came to be." Since that time, New York's disabilities programs have "gone on to enrich the lives of hundreds of thousands of New Yorkers," but, the text reminds viewers, "Willowbrook continues to demonstrate the need to strengthen the service delivery system." Willowbrook serves as a constant reminder to improve services for those with developmental disabilities, and because of that, "on this solemn occasion, we must remember not only the progress that has been made, but also how this journey began."

At its start, the outline offers a much broader sense of history than the monuments on the CSI campus, but it still creates monumental heroes. While multiple individuals and groups advocated for the developmentally disabled group, those actions culminate in Rivera's journalism and in the creation of a state agency. Additionally, the timeline does not foreclose the past in the same way as the CSI monuments. The opening text places viewers in a relationship to the past, as memory of Willowbrook reminds people why improved care for the developmentally disabled is needed, but part of that memory is the monumental recognition of "progress that has been made." Witnessing the past is not foreclosed, but rather than focus on injustice as is the norm for witnessing and for memorials, viewers are called to witness and celebrate the progress of the state in caring for the developmentally disabled.

The next display begins the timeline in 1938 and focuses on the early efforts to appropriate money for the school and find a suitable site on Staten Island. The site, the display notes, was coopted by the federal government for a military hospital during World War II. The images here include maps of the area; drawings of buildings on the site, including what would become known as Building 2; pictures of men at the military hospital; and newspaper clippings about the plans for Willowbrook and the closing of the military hospital.

The story of the Willowbrook School proper begins on the next display board, which initiates an *incrementum,* or series, describing the decline and increasing squalor of the school. It begins in 1952 with the school's opening, noting that "by the end of the year, the census is 2450." For almost every year marked on the timeline from this point, the census of residents is noted. The figure of 2,450 increases to 2,887, then 3,406, on upwards to 6,201. The images and newspaper clippings in the three display boards leading to Rivera's exposé on Willowbrook visualize the increasingly squalid conditions. The display board on the school's opening depicts active children dressed in everyday clothes and engaged in a variety of activities. One or more female nurses or aides are shown in almost every image. On the next display board, the majority of patients shown are in hospital gowns. Some lie in bed with their limbs contorted and their gowns in disarray. A group of African American children are shown helping one another up the stairs in one image and crouching, unattended, on the floor by a door in another. An image of a large ward shows men in various stages of dress and undress with one or two aides in the background, and alongside these images is a newspaper clipping with the headline "Retarded in Overcrowded Institutions." In the third, patients are either undressed or in torn and damaged clothing. Another image shows an infant in a crib indistinguishable from a cage, while a headline that appears to have been torn from a newspaper observes, "Willowbrook: No Bed of Roses."

The negative trend of increasing population and decreasing quality of care reaches its culmination in the fourth display, titled "The Scandal." It opens with this observation: "Designed for a maximum capacity of 4000 people, by 1965 the population had grown to more than 6000." It continues by noting the school had become "a hotbed of scandal and controversy," and "one significant controversy included the nearly 20 years of medical study of hepatitis, during which children were intentionally infected in order to identify possible cures." After referencing Krugman's studies, the display mentions Robert Kennedy's declaration that Willowbrook was a "snakepit" and then a series of articles in the *Staten Island Advance* that were critical of the school. It then introduces Geraldo Rivera's exposé on Willowbrook, "which led to a national outcry over the quality of care and lack of rights for people with developmental disabilities."

The timeline portion of "The Scandal" display board acts as the inflection point where care for the developmentally disabled improves. The report on Willowbrook's population disappears. The only numerical report on this display come from 1967: "20,000 individuals with developmental disabilities reside in 20 institutions across New York State." The most prominent image on "The Scandal" display board is a picture taken of Geraldo Rivera and his camera crew, cropped and enlarged from a picture of the men right before their initial clandestine visit to Willowbrook in January 1972.[40] The next largest images are clippings from newspapers: one reports on Robert Kennedy's remarks about Willowbrook; another is a headline from the *Staten Island Advance,* "Willowbrook: Inside the Cages"; and the third is an advertisement for Rivera's extended documentary *Willowbrook: The Last Great Disgrace,* which opens with the line "Tonight, as a public service, we're going to make you sick." Journalism, especially the work of Rivera, is framed as the impetus for change at Willowbrook that brings to light "the stories of neglect, abuse, and more" referenced in the opening display.

In addition to the heroic framing of Rivera, the Scandal display is noteworthy as the *only* reference to Krugman's hepatitis experiments in official public memory. Furthermore, while Krugman's research ran for more than twenty years, as the display notes, the timeline only flags the hepatitis research for the years 1963–1966. This is accompanied by the descriptions "controversial medical studies are conducted" and "public outcry forces the study to cease." What is not made clear is that the research continued past 1966, and it is also unclear from the timeline why these three years are noteworthy. Those familiar with the study might recognize that this is the period where children were being enrolled in

Krugman's study and admitted to Willowbrook while general admission (e.g., admissions that did not require submitting to research) were halted, creating concerns about consent and coercion.

The four display boards appearing after "The Scandal" initiate a new incrementum away from the squalor and overpopulation toward fewer large institutions and better care in community settings, reversing the incrementum of the exhibit's first half. The most prominent images in the two display boards after "The Scandal" emphasize the destruction of Willowbrook's iconic Building 2. The display frames the destruction as the beginning of improvement. This is reinforced by the newspaper clippings and images showing officials signing papers that start the close of the school and the reform of New York's care of the developmentally disabled. In the next display, titled "The Closure," the text discusses the Willowbrook Consent Decree that led to the school's closure. It notes, "The Willowbrook Decree was signed, committing New York to improve opportunities for community placement for those residing at Willowbrook" and it "helped usher in the expansive community residential system in place today." The linguistic framing is notable: The decree is the active agent, "committing" people to action and "helping" create the system in place today. The signing of the decree occurs in passive voice. Given that the decree was essentially a capitulation by New York State to parents suing it over their children's living conditions, these shifts in voice deflect attention from memories of litigious confrontation into a recognition and celebration of the state's current system, which is framed as marked improvement.

Images of the school's destruction and description of the consent decree open the new incrementum, which begins with the observation that at the time of Building 2's demolition, "11,798 people live in development centers; 12,000 people live in the community." The timeline now highlights the diminution of Willowbrook's population: Where the increase in population implied a decreased quality of life, the reduction in population implies an improvement in the quality of life for those with developmental disabilities, which culminates in the observation for 1987 that "Willowbrook is declared officially and forever closed." This incrementum is discursively continued in the timeline's observation that year after year more development centers are closed and more people with developmental disabilities live in the community, a conclusion reinforced in the headline for the penultimate display—"Building a Better System." The closing visual images offer a marked contrast from the images of squalor in the first four displays and the images of demolition that inaugurate the new incrementum. The display boards depict people with developmental disabilities engaged in recreational activities and interacting with others in community settings. In every image, they are smiling. The contrast of these smiling faces to the images of squalor brings the traveling exhibit's incrementum to its culmination.

The "Remembering Willowbrook" traveling exhibit articulates a memory that valorizes both OPWDD and the work of Geraldo Rivera. Rivera's journalism acts as the display's pivot, where the timeline shifts from a downward trajectory of overcrowding and worsening conditions to a trajectory of decreased population at Willowbrook and improved conditions for the developmentally disabled everywhere in the state. That improvement is made possible and safeguarded by the state, whose "progress" in caring for the developmentally disabled is to be witnessed and honored by viewers. While the exhibit does not have the nakedly monumental qualities of the permanent memory work at Willowbrook/CSI and it does remember the squalor in which Willowbrook's residents lived, the exhibit ultimately reinforces the permanent memory work's consignment of Willowbrook's squalor to a past that has been superseded.

The exhibit also downplays present concerns about care for the developmentally disabled. The depiction of improved conditions is interwoven with bureaucratic language of "service delivery systems" and "person-centered services" emphasizing the role of OPWDD and its community housing programs in enabling this upward trajectory. Yet, such language deflects attention from persistent problems in the care of the developmentally disabled, even when those issues are mentioned. For example, the timeline notes that in 2011, "the *New York Times* begins a yearlong series focusing on abuse of people with developmental disabilities and other system breakdowns. OPWDD launches one of the most significant reform initiatives in its history." While the display recognizes the existence of ongoing challenges in caring for the developmentally disabled, the issue is downplayed overall. That reference to the *New York Times*'s stories is placed in the middle of the display board's timeline, and it shares the year 2011 with a longer, detailed account of the anniversary of the Americans with Disabilities Act and the closure of a developmental center. Ongoing issues of neglect are minimized while past issues of neglect are sequestered from the present by Rivera's exposé and the "scandal" that ensued.[41]

Overall, the exhibit retains many aspects of monumental form and "minimal remembrance." The exhibit *does* offer more didactic content, but the story is still one of triumph. Journalists reveal scandals, which are resolved by the state. While the conditions at Willowbrook offer visitors to the exhibit a warning about neglecting the developmentally disabled, it is a warning that steadily recedes into the past as institutionalization dwindles away. What is occluded, if not completely forgotten, in this memory work is that the very state portrayed as fixing the problems created the problems in the first place and still has issues and problems in how it organizes care for the developmentally disabled today. This official memory work differs markedly from the memories offered by non-state actors.

Vernacular Memory

Unlike the official, institutional practices of minimal remembrance, vernacular or lay memories of Willowbrook lack a material form like the monuments on Willowbrook/CSI's campus. Yet, multiple memories are produced about the school, and a search of the Internet for "Willowbrook" will produce numerous results, in addition to journalistic accounts of the school.[42] These vernacular memories urge people to remember Willowbrook the school or Willowbrook the experiment as a bulwark against the dehumanization of the developmentally disabled and the institutionalization that enabled it. Most vernacular memory work draws heavily from Rivera's exposé, using images of the school's squalor to animate the memory work with disgust and anger. As Blair and colleagues note, the potent public feelings invoked facilitate *philia* as witnesses to Willowbrook's horror. Attention is focused on the school as a whole. These public feelings direct attention away from the hepatitis experiments toward the conditions that facilitated those experiments. Yet articulating different images of Willowbrook shifts the affective basis for philia and allows for different types of memory, specifically a consideration of Krugman's hepatitis experiments. Two contrasting instances of public memory illustrate this dynamic: the 1997 documentary *Unforgotten: 25 Years after Willowbrook* and the 2012 short film *Willowbrook.* These performances of memory—one a documentary of family experiences with the school, the other a "based on true events" fictional account of the hepatitis experiments—draw on the mnestic capacity of language to position audiences as witnesses to different aspects of the school's history.

UNFORGOTTEN: 25 YEARS AFTER WILLOWBROOK

Many vernacular memories emphasize the horrors of Willowbrook and how they should never have occurred. This message and the implied solution are most fully articulated in the documentary *Unforgotten,* released on the twenty-fifth anniversary of Geraldo Rivera's exposé. It uses the stories of four families as the vehicle to explore Willowbrook and the aftermath of institutionalization. *Unforgotten* takes the form of a standard expository documentary. Narrator Danny Aiello and the family members recount events from institutional and personal histories, and the visuals provide "evidence" for the claims verbalized. The expository documentary's emphasis on realism and its familiarity vouchsafe the stories provided (i.e., they are true or real).[43] In doing so, the documentary grounds the experiences of the family, especially the non-disabled family, as the appropriate locus for understanding Willowbrook and recognizing the humanity of the developmentally disabled.

The families' stories begin during the documentary's opening credits. They emphasize the emotional shock of discovering one's child was developmentally disabled as well as the ignorance surrounding disability in the mid-twentieth century. The families of Sal Giordano, Margaret Goodman, Patty Ann Meskell, and Luis Rivera tell the stories of when they discovered that their family member had a developmental disability. Margaret Goodman's mother says, "Finally, the doctor told me Margaret was mentally retarded, and I didn't understand what that was." Sal Giordano's father describes his emotional trauma at discovering that his son was developmentally disabled, and his mother describes how they wanted to keep him at home but were unable to do so. One of Patty Ann Meskell's sisters observed, "In the Fifties, you didn't keep them at home. You sent them away. Your family encouraged it. The priest encouraged it. The doctor told you to do it."

After establishing that these families committed a member to Willowbrook, the documentary fades into a medium-shot image of narrator Danny Aiello, who observes, "The horror stories of the Willowbrook State School are now history, but many of the survivors and their families are very much alive today." The documentary then returns to the family stories to expand on Aiello's point. Families recount the smell of urine and feces and the random moans and screams that would punctuate their visits to Willowbrook. They also recounted the emotional toll that came from having a family member in Willowbrook. Patty Ann's sister, Katie Meskell, who was an executive producer for the documentary, remembered seeing the same families riding the bus to Willowbrook every week, but they "never talked to each other because of the shame." Luis Rivera's oldest brother notes, "It was a struggle, and it was a painful struggle. . . . Simply because he's not at home with us anymore didn't mean we didn't care. Simply because he can't—because he's not able to speak doesn't mean he doesn't have anything to say."

The documentary returns to Aiello, who notes that many might only recall Willowbrook vaguely, "but for those who lived there, it was a day-to-day struggle to survive." The video then cuts to film from Rivera's investigative report on Willowbrook. Over images of the neglect at the

Willowbrook School, Aiello intones, "Life at Willowbrook held no ex-
pectations. It was endless days with nothing to do and no one to talk
to." As the images continue, Aiello observes that few children went to
classes, despite Willowbrook being called a school; that the patient to
staff ratio in 1972 was thirty to one; and that all residents would contract
hepatitis within six months of admission. Families again offer testimony
of the harms experienced by their children and siblings at the school.
The families' stories of neglect and the images from the documentary are
reaffirmed by Geraldo Rivera and former resident Bernard Carabello,
who flatly declares, "It was like living in hell; it was like living in a concentration camp."

After the interview segment with Carabello, the documentary offers a series of images of a dilapidated building from the Willowbrook
campus. As that series fades out, Aiello notes, "Many people assume the
human stories from Willowbrook ended when the institution was forced
to close its doors. In fact, that was only the beginning." *Unforgotten* then
begins presenting the stories of Patty Ann Meskell and Luis Rivera's
families in greater detail. Each segment combines historical film and
photos with film of the family in the present. The contemporary images
always include all members of the family, especially the developmentally disabled family member, and discussions of the psychological and
emotional toll of the separation and neglect inflicted at Willowbrook.
After describing these two families in detail, the documentary returns
to Aiello, who tells viewers, "The last twenty-five years have brought a
lot of changes. Many institutions such as Willowbrook have, through
public pressure, litigation, and government reform, been phased out in
favor of home care, group homes, alternative forms of education, and
social integration." It then describes Meskell, Rivera, and Carabello's
lives, including the facts that Patty Ann Meskell has a boyfriend, Luis's
family no longer feels like they are treated as visitors with no say in Luis's
care, and Carabello has a role on state committees monitoring care for
the developmentally disabled.

The documentary then culminates in scenes from the Special Olympics. Aiello announces, "Undoubtedly the public consciousness has

been raised over the past several decades. The Special Olympics with representatives from over seventy countries around the world is a testament, a powerful demonstration of renewed priorities." The families featured in the documentary, along with Geraldo Rivera and Bernard Carabello, affirm the "testament" of the Special Olympics. For example, Luis Rivera's older brother says, "Willowbrook taught me that they were first human beings and then disabled." Katie Meskell encapsulates the documentary's message: "Willowbrook was much more than an institution. It was an attitude, an attitude of disrespect for people with handicapping conditions, and it can easily happen again if we turn our backs on these folks." The overt goal of *Unforgotten* is to foster memory and act as a bulwark against forgetting the horror of Willowbrook. In remembering the institution, it evokes disgust and horror at the conditions at the school by repeating the images from the Rivera exposé and supplementing them with testimony from the families of former residents. It then identifies two attitudes as the reason Willowbrook's residents were neglected: disrespect for the developmentally disabled and a failure to acknowledge their humanity and consubstantiality with those who are developmentally typical. Framing the "problem" as an attitude of disrespect universalizes the message of the documentary.

Unforgotten calls audiences to witness Willowbrook as a metonymy for disrespect and a lack of acknowledgment. Medicine demands care for others—care that is sorely lacking at Willowbrook. The documentary highlights this to craft bioethical memory. The school's squalor and any disgust viewers feel not only create solidarity in the viewers' collective role as witnesses but also foster a sense of the *unheimlich*. If the problem is one of disrespect, then individuals are called to account for the ways in which they might have disrespected the developmentally disabled. The solution, then, is both simple and rhetorically powerful: one acknowledges the humanity of others, especially the developmentally disabled. As Michael Hyde argues, acknowledgment is in many ways an ideal outcome of experiences of the unheimlich.[44] The documentary resolves that experience of the unheimlich by offering the Special Olympics as the scene of acknowledgment. The use of the Special Olympics in

Unforgotten partakes of the "relentless positivity" that other scholars have observed in media coverage of the event.[45] Rhetorically, this relentless positivity balances the horror of Willowbrook displayed earlier in the documentary, resolving the disquiet of the uncanny with the positivity of acknowledging the developmentally disabled.

While powerful, the rhetorical performance of acknowledgment as the apotheosis of Willowbrook's bioethical memory is rhetorically, ethically, and historically problematic. The documentary's use of the Special Olympics emphasizes disability as an ethical test.[46] The "correct" answer to that test is what Rosemarie Garland Thomson calls a rhetoric of sentimentality, the evocation of pity accomplished ultimately by diminishing the developmentally disabled.[47] The focus on individual acknowledgment translates into a priority for individuals in their interactions with others, but prioritizing individual action is problematic as the challenge represented by institutions like Willowbrook is collective and political. The documentary's call for people to "respect" the developmentally disabled obscures *how* Willowbrook happened. It obscures the drive toward institutionalized care across the nineteenth century and first two-thirds of the twentieth century, followed by the trend toward deinstitutionalization since the early 1970s.[48] In the United States, care for the developmentally disabled has been either a local- or state-level issue, but states and municipalities must address a variety of issues. Those who advocate for the developmentally disabled must compete with other groups in their attempts to influence state budgets and see their priorities recognized and funded. In the post–World War II era, states were encouraged to invest heavily in *building institutions* but not in staffing and maintaining them, a dynamic not captured by *Unforgotten's* calls for recognition and respect.[49] The focus on individual acknowledgment also obscures the present consequences of deinstitutionalization, a process that the documentary praises. While the developmentally disabled are no longer warehoused in state schools and mental institutions, all too many are either homeless or in jails.[50] The money needed to provide care for many developmentally and mentally disabled individuals at the level they might require is not provided by state or federal coffers, and given the cost and scale required, all too many people balk at expanding systems of care, despite accepting the call to respect the developmentally disabled.

Additionally, the documentary's emphasis on family limits the scope of care and activism. The structure of the entire documentary articulates the family as the key site for acknowledging and respecting the developmentally disabled. The documentary's realism also provides the family narrative's further credence by amplifying the sense that the family members know what is best for developmentally disabled family members. The emphasis on "normalization" in care for the developmentally disabled makes the emphasis on family logical. Yet, it also places the obligation of care solely on families. For some families, this is an obligation that they will have the resources to absorb, but for many families, the costs of care in terms of their time and financial resources will be quite high. Additionally, framing the family as the site of recognition and care risks disempowering advocates and caregivers who are not family members and disempowering those developmentally disabled individuals who would advocate for themselves. Here again, the structure and content of the documentary reinforces this trend. The documentary begins and ends with family members speaking on behalf of the developmentally disabled. Only two of the disabled individuals at the center of *Unforgotten*'s story appear outside of photographs: Patty Ann Meskell and Luis Rivera. Rivera is incapable of speech or independent movement. Meskell can speak but does so very little in the documentary, and other sources indicate that she faces substantial challenges in speaking.[51] While these individuals might be representative of the former population of Willowbrook, the choice to focus on them fosters an image of developmental disability that does not include self-advocacy.[52]

WILLOWBROOK

The majority of vernacular memory work on Willowbrook focuses on the conditions at the school and foregoes remembering the scientific research to which some of its residents were subjected. One notable exception is

Ross Cohen's award-winning 2012 short film *Willowbrook*. The film is a fictionalized account, "based on true events" as an opening text insert informs viewers. Dramatized accounts of historical events are often a source of historical information for the American public, and "they afford a means through which uncomfortable histories can be smoothed over, retold, and ascribed new meanings."[53] Fiction has a capacity for crafting public and bioethical memory. *Willowbrook* depicts the challenges of both practicing medicine and conducting medical research, and it highlights the tension between empathy for patients and the medical practitioner's need for clinical distance in order to perform medical care and medical research. In order to accomplish this meditation on medical practice, it has to sanitize both Willowbrook *and* the details of Krugman's research in order to deflect public feelings of horror and disgust while allowing viewers to foster a sense of the unheimlich and reflect on medical research and moral obligations toward others.

Willowbrook tells the story of Bill Huntsman, a first-year resident who in 1964 joins the medical team of Dr. Horowitz, the film's proxy for Saul Krugman. Huntsman learns that his primary job will be injecting new patients on Horowitz's research ward with MS1, the strain of hepatitis Horowitz has isolated. Bill faces this troubling task in short order, as Mrs. Sussman considers whether to admit her son Brian to the research ward, the only part of Willowbrook admitting new patients.[54] Bill, after a surreal dialogue with the otherwise uncommunicative Brian, calls Mrs. Sussman and urges her not to admit her son. The next morning, after passing Mrs. Sussman in the hallway, Bill encounters Dr. Horowitz, who orders him to administer the injection to Brian. Despite his obvious emotional distress, Bill does so.

Throughout, the film attenuates the horror produced by the conditions at Willowbrook and in the experiments. Typically, the horror experienced at witnessing the neglect of Willowbrook's patients, which is made present by the consistent reuse of film from Geraldo Rivera's exposé, overwhelms consideration of Krugman's work. When we see again developmentally disabled children left to flounder naked in disease and filth, the issue of medical research effectively pales so much that it disappears. *Willowbrook* attenuates the affective force of the neglect by sanitizing the conditions at the school. In the opening scene, we see Brian Sussman in a wheelchair in a room by himself; he has the luxury of his own space, is not crammed into a room with others. In a later scene, Dr. Horowitz is showing Bill Huntsman one of Willowbrook's general wards. As they walk, the camera shows Bill noticing a number of young boys in the rooms of the ward. The rooms are occupied by eight to ten boys. They make unintelligible noises and contort their bodies in awkward poses or roll on the floor. Their clothes are unbuttoned and several lack a shirt. Over these images, Horowitz describes the conditions at Willowbrook: "The general ward was built to accommodate four thousand residents. Current enrollment is over six thousand. Disease spreads easily. Infections, dysentery, parasites, and the ever-present hepatitis." The film offers a depiction of the conditions at Willowbrook: the images of developmentally disabled boys in various degrees of undress and neglect are combined with Horowitz's exposition to frame the conditions in which the hepatitis research occurred. Yet these images and words—for all their depiction of neglect—fall short of the affective power created by images from the actual Willowbrook, where many children were naked, some were bound with torn strips and remnants of their clothes to prevent them from hurting themselves or others, and where the sounds of their moans overwhelmed the recording equipment used by Rivera and his camera crew, creating haunting reverberations. The sensory combination found in the recordings of the Willowbrook School overwhelm; the sensory combinations found in the film *Willowbrook* contextualize, rendering intelligible the actions in the remainder of the film.

The film also attenuates the horror of the experiment by depicting infection with hepatitis as the result of injection. Two scenes of infection are shown, one near the beginning of the film and the other in the closing scene of the film. Yet, in the actual experiments, hepatitis was introduced through *ingestion:* children were infected with hepatitis by placing infected stool in food. Portraying children consuming feces-laden chocolate milk would produce strong visceral reactions. Hypodermic needles, by contrast, might make some nervous, but they are an unremarkable component of clinical settings. Their commonplace quality makes them useful as a tool for symbolizing medical practice while also attenuating affective responses.[55]

Second, the film opens the space for experiencing the feeling of the uncanny and acknowledging the developmentally disabled Other through a fantasia of Brian Sussman as an articulate young man.[56] This fantastic element of the story appears in the opening scene, and it operates in what Rosemarie Garland Thomson describes as a rhetoric of the wondrous, imbuing the disabled individual with divine or superhuman qualities.[57] As the film fades into a scene of falling snow, Brian says in a voice-over,

> I have this plan for what I'd do if I could control the weather. I'd grow the tree in the back so high it'd be ten times the size of the building. Then, the sky would open up, and it'd snow. A thick, wet snow. Take a day of that, maybe two. The oak's boughs would finally bend under the weight, like those old-time petticoats. I can see it so clear in my mind how beautiful it could be.

As the last remark is offered, the film cuts to a close-up of Brian's face, and in that moment, the film leaves the fantasy of the articulate, imaginative Brian Sussman. The background music abruptly ends, and in the silence, we see the disabled Brian who cannot speak or move and who remains unresponsive as two aides move him from the wheelchair in which he was sitting to his bed. During the voice-over, the film shows us the snow and the oversized trees summoned by Brian's imagined powers, but with the cut to the film's mundane reality, those disappear alongside Brian's words.

The fantasia appears a second time after Bill struggles indecisively with his conscience over the work he must perform. He stands in the doorway to Brian's room:

BILL: How did you get out of bed?
BRIAN: I flew.

BILL: (*stunned, as he had not expected an answer*) What??

BRIAN: I'm kidding. [*BILL slowly enters room.*] I'm not very funny. Think you'd be funny? Locked up all this time?

Bill and Brian engage in a conversation. Brian tells Bill, "I've had this idea that if I focus—really focus with my mind—that someone'll hear what I'm thinking." Later in the conversation, Bill asks Brian what he wants people to hear, and Brian answers, "I guess just, 'I'm alive.'" With that admission, the fantasia ends, signaled by the abrupt stop of the background music and a sudden jump cut from a close-up of Bill kneeling in front of Brian talking to Bill standing in the entrance to the room, with Brian again nonresponsive, spittle dripping down his chin, in the foreground. The fantasia returns briefly a third time at the close of the film as Bill administers the hepatitis injection to Brian. This time, the camera assumes Brian's point of view, showing the needle injecting the MS-1 hepatitis strain into Brian's arm. Brian's opening monologue about controlling the weather can again be heard in voice-over. As the monologue continues, the camera then pans up to a close-up of Bill's face, showing his conflicted feelings about his own actions. In the background, snow is falling.

The first two scenes depict Brian as articulate, allowing the audience to enter his imagination as he controls the weather, and then allowing Bill (and the audience along with him) to talk with Brian and know he is aware and articulate behind or inside the disabled body. Finally, the audience takes on Brian's point of view as he is injected with hepatitis. These moments utilize the rhetoric of the wondrous, less to "secure the ordinariness of the viewer," as Garland Thomson argues, but to craft a space, however problematic, for acknowledgment and identification.[58] Each moment offers the audience identification with the fantasia of a developmentally disabled individual, whose articulate soul is trapped in a recalcitrant body that prevents him from pleading for the acknowledgment he wants and deserves. Yet these images exist alongside the inarticulate Brian Sussman. The two images jar with one another, as reflected in the abrupt transitions between the two. *Willowbrook* makes Brian Sussman, and thus all developmentally disabled people, live in the eyes of

Bill Huntsman and in the eyes of the audience, but it does not let them live and be acknowledged as they are. By choosing the most abject and incommunicative disabled body to represent all those at Willowbrook who were disabled, the film fantasizes the possibility of communication, deflecting attention from the possibility of communication with those who are developmentally disabled as they are in the flesh and not our imaginations.

Ultimately, Bill's acknowledgment of Brian's humanity does not prevent the hepatitis injection. Bill's emotional trauma does not stop him from putting the needle in Brian's arm. Bill's attempt to act on his acknowledgment of Brian's humanity—his phone call the night before to Brian's mother—has failed, leaving Bill with no other option. It is here that the importance of Dr. Horowitz's character to the story comes into sharp relief. He performs the role of the experienced clinician, who blends empathy for Bill and for Mrs. Sussman with detachment from the conditions of children at Willowbrook. This role reflects the recognition that conditions at the school were difficult to change, and the willingness of medical researchers to take advantage of that situation.

Horowitz's experience and detachment are performed alongside Bill Huntsman's naiveté and engagement. Horowitz's experience is first highlighted during his description of the conditions at Willowbrook. As he is talking, he walks down the hallway past the young boys in the general ward, who are partially dressed, moaning, and spilling out into the hallway. Horowitz steps over the boys, not once looking at them, while Huntsman goes out of his way to avoid stepping over or on them. The conditions in Willowbrook's general wards do not shock or surprise Horowitz; he is able to walk over and around the children in the wards. Horowitz's emotional detachment is also displayed during the scene where he asks Brian's mother to enroll him in the research ward. She asks to see him, and Dr. Horowitz encourages her to *not* see Brian. After she insists, Brian is brought into the room and sits unresponsive in a wheelchair. His mother leans in toward Brian and turns his head to look into his eyes. While Bill Huntsman stares intently at the interaction, Horowitz averts his gaze. A moment later Horowitz tells Mrs. Sussman,

"I know this is hard. There is a part of you that wants him home. That's natural. It's the maternal instinct. That's a good thing, but it's . . . indiscriminate. It leads us to moor down things best set to sea." Throughout this scene, Horowitz encourages Brian's mother to avoid engaging with Brian and experiencing attachment and acknowledgment. On one level, in the face of the inevitable need to leave a child at the school, Horowitz is encouraging her to minimize her own emotional suffering, but he is also adding a new individual to his research program. When faced with the moment where Mrs. Sussman looks into Brian's face seeking some acknowledgment from her nonresponsive son, he averts his eyes. He performs the detachment he advocates for others. This clinical detachment is to some degree necessary for medical professionals to successfully perform their role, but here, it leads Horowitz to treat the children in his ward solely as raw material for research.

Horowitz's view of the children and what can and ought to be done to them is articulated in the closing scene of the film. Bill Huntsman enters an examination room to find Brian being secured to an examination table by two nurses while Horowitz watches. After seeing that Mrs. Sussman has signed the consent form, Bill protests:

> BILL: But there's no benefit to these children.
>
> HOROWITZ: This isn't about these children. It's about the future. Finding a vaccine for people at risk, whether they be patients on the ward or boys in uniform. We need to keep going.
>
> BILL: Don't tell me you think he'd be better off in the general ward? [*Silence.*]
>
> HOROWITZ: We have supplies here. Medicine. This is the best Brian Sussman can do, and if the price is 4cc's of MS1, then you know what? [*Abrupt sound of arm restraint being pulled tight on Brian Sussman.*] That's the price.
>
> HOROWITZ: (*gently*) Administer the injection.

In Horowitz's view, the only good option for developmentally disabled individuals like Brian Sussman is placement in the research ward; but that placement comes at the cost of infection with hepatitis. Horowitz performs a ratiocinative attitude toward Brian, discounting the issue of benefits to the individual and the individual's dignity when compared to the potential benefits to society. He also shows concern for Bill's emotional struggle as he faces having to inject Brian with the hepatitis virus.

Willowbrook uses a fictionalized vehicle to allow the audience to witness the hepatitis experiments conducted at the Willowbrook School. The film downplays the extent of Willowbrook's squalor in order to focus attention on the hepatitis experiments. Audiences witness the complexities of clinical care and medical research. In doing so, the film fosters the unheimlich, as medical care and research become strange and unfamiliar. It also highlights the limitations of the unheimlich for medical practice, noted in chapter 2. For medical professionals who are trained to practice clinical detachment or detached concern, the experience of the unheimlich might be interpreted as troublesome doubts undermining one's ability to provide care and conduct research. The film positions audiences at this pivot point between doubt and contemplation in order to consider the injustices of the hepatitis experiments and how they can act in the present to address the experiments' legacy. The film also highlights the limits of acknowledgment without broader structural support for acting on that acknowledgment, complicating the ethical vision found in memory work like *Unforgotten*. Bill Huntsman acknowledges the humanity of Brian Sussman, but only in the space of the fantasia, and he fails to prevent Brian from being infected with hepatitis. The film does not even address the possibility that Bill Huntsman could walk away from Willowbrook, in part because such a move by a first-year resident would be unlikely and would not prevent Brian Sussman's infection.

The Willowbrook Mile and the
(Im)possibility of a Unified Memory Culture

Memory of Willowbrook is ultimately a bioethical memory: It witnesses the multiple ways in which those with developmental disabilities suffered at a school intended for their long-term medical care. Their suffering was terrible, and the documentation of it by Geraldo Rivera and a small film crew has a great deal of affective power. Yet not all memory work about the school depicts that suffering. The affective power of that suffering often prompts a powerful impulse toward minimal remembrance. When the closure and deinstitutionalization process was complete, the State of New York had no desire to recall its role in allowing Willowbrook's squalor or its foot-dragging in ending those conditions. To achieve that minimal remembrance, official memory work employs a monumental form. History is reformed into a heroic narrative, and a great deal of the past is elided. The state is lauded for improving conditions for developmentally disabled people across the state, even as the memorials elide the state's culpability for the horrible conditions of the school. Visitors to the various plaques and the traveling exhibit about the school are called to witness heroic actions, whether it is the state alone or the state in conjunction with the work of Geraldo Rivera to expose Willowbrook's conditions. In creating this heroic narrative, conditions at the school are downplayed, either by being ignored outright, or by being framed as existing solely in the past with little or no relevance for the present day. Here the witnessing that bioethical memory demands is twisted into a celebration of a fictionalized actor: a heroic state ending conditions, while ignoring the state's very culpability for what it ends.

Much of the vernacular memory, as represented by the documentary *Unforgotten,* makes greater use of Rivera's exposé but contrasts it with images from the Special Olympics. The footage of Willowbrook's conditions is meant to encourage feelings of disgust and the unheimlich as individuals contemplate the degree to which they neglected or ignored those with developmental disabilities. That sense of disorientation and the uncanny at the sight of institutionalized neglect is resolved through acknowledging and respecting the developmentally disabled, as symbolized by the Special Olympics. Yet, this resolution fails to address the social and political challenges of providing care, replacing that with individual acknowledgment of humanity as the solution.

Finally, *Willowbrook* of all the memory artifacts studied shifts attention away from the conditions at the school to more directly face the ethical issues of the hepatitis experiments conducted at Willowbrook by Saul Krugman. The film's fictionalized account uses fantasia to create a sense of the uncanny. The goal is an ethical contemplation of research and clinical detachment. Audiences witness the challenges that the main character, Bill Huntsman, faces and can consider how to best address the injustices of this research today. In many ways, the film dovetails with the version of Willowbrook in disciplinary bioethics's origin story: Willowbrook is a warning about consent and the rights of the developmentally disabled in research. To facilitate this memory work, the film must minimize the elements of the school and the experiment that evoke disgust.

All of these bioethical memory artifacts position audiences in relation to a powerfully moving set of images from the school's past. Official memory work engages in minimal remembrance to lock these images away in the past. Most vernacular memory employs it to reaffirm the need to acknowledge the humanity of the developmentally disabled. Memory work devoted to remembering Krugman's experiments must attenuate those images; it is only when the affective power of Willowbrook's squalor is downplayed that remembrance of Krugman's experiments gain purchase. Against this complicated interplay of different articulations of memory, we should consider attempts to expand the memory artifacts at the Willowbrook campus. On September 14, 2016, the College of Staten Island held a groundbreaking for the Willowbrook Mile, a walking trail consisting of ten different memory stations developed in coordination between CSI, OPWDD, and the Institute for Basic Research in Developmental Disabilities.[59] Two of the stops would be the already existing monuments on CSI's campus—the Building 19 memorial and the 1987 commemorative plaque. The current proposal for the memory stations will include audiovisual materials, as well as materials in Braille. None of it has been built, and plans for memory stations have been scaled back substantially.

The development of the Mile has been a slow process. When I first visited CSI in early 2015, the Mile was supposed to have been built, but no ground had been broken. During the groundbreaking for the Mile, assemblyman Michael Cusick said that community groups had been pushing for the Mile for over a decade.[60] The most recent version does briefly reference Krugman's experiments, but an early version of the proposal from 2015 did not include any references to the hepatitis experiments. Even as more material is developed, the proposed Mile incorporates wholesale the monumental memory work that already exists on the CSI campus. The tensions between the three strands of memory highlighted above make the attempts to unify these memories in the construct of the Willowbrook Mile challenging. Those challenges have taken years to resolve, and even with the groundbreaking, the memory work of the Mile is still relatively unformed. How much the impulses of the vernacular groups will hold sway and how much a monumental form of history will prevail remains to be seen. While minimal remembrance shaped official memory of Willowbrook, the growing temporal distance from the school and the legal battles around implementing the consent decree might lead to less minimal remembrance as plans for the Willowbrook Mile are implemented. A radically different situation can be found with a public memory in Cincinnati for a series of radiation experiments that were contemporaneous with Willowbrook and Tuskegee but have been deliberately forgotten multiple times.

CHAPTER 5

Attempting to Forget

THE UNIVERSITY OF CINCINNATI RADIATION STUDIES

———•◆•———

I n October 1971, public attention focused on radiologist Dr. Eugene Saenger and the University of Cincinnati (UC). For eleven years, Saenger had been under contract with the Department of Defense (DOD) to study radiation's effects on humans—specifically to identify a possible "biological dosimeter" for assessing how much radiation a soldier had received. Such a dosimeter, if it could be found, would be immensely valuable to the DOD in a nuclear war.[1] To identify such a dosimeter, Saenger and his research team exposed patients with metastatic cancers (i.e., cancers that had spread throughout the body) to 100–300 rads of Cobalt-60 radiation. Such doses were considered dangerous, if not fatal, for healthy humans.[2] Saenger and his team refused to give patients medication to prevent nausea because they wanted to assess when nausea would occur after radiation exposure. For the first seven years, patients were not given any treatment to counteract the depletion of red and white blood cells the radiation would cause. In the eighth year, Saenger and his colleagues started an additional experiment involving the (at the time, new) practice of removing and then reinfusing bone marrow.

News reports on Saenger's work brought the scrutiny of Senator Edward Kennedy (D-MA) and Senator Mike Gravel (D-AK). Their initial investigations and demand for answers about the project led to two reports by University of Cincinnati faculty, a report from the American College of Radiologists, an opinion from the General Accounting Office, and multiple news stories. But then, the story suddenly disappeared. Kennedy dropped the issue, and the University of Cincinnati quietly dropped the DOD contract. Saenger's research—and all the public attention to it—ended with a whimper and not a bang.[3]

In 1993, Department of Energy secretary Hazel O'Leary announced that human radiation experiments had been conducted by the federal government from the late 1940s through the 1970s.[4] Stories about the radiation studies conducted in Cincinnati began circulating again, along with stories of other radiation experiments. This led to multiple congressional hearings and the creation of President Bill Clinton's Advisory Committee on Human Radiation Experiments (ACHRE), headed by bioethicist Ruth Faden. The families of the cancer patients also sued Saenger and the University of Cincinnati, and the lawsuit was settled out of court. The settlement led to the creation of a memorial on the grounds of the University of Cincinnati's University Hospital. Yet, despite this attention, many in Cincinnati and elsewhere are still unaware of these events. Undergraduate students are shocked and surprised when I tell them that such an experiment happened at their university. Faculty, staff, and trainees at UC's medical center are equally unaware of it.

The Whole Body Radiation Study (WBS)[5] at the University of Cincinnati represents a case of *meaningful forgetting*, where the capacity to create and sustain public and bioethical memories of the event has been undermined. Meaningful forgetting is an intensification of minimal remembrance, and it is facilitated by *philia*, specifically the affiliation of physicians to a specific concord or vision of themselves and medical research. It consists of rhetorically significant actions and contexts that render memory contents absent or undermine their circulation.[6]

Forgetting the Cincinnati WBS study—by impairing how the story of the WBS study circulated—was valuable and rhetorically significant for both Senator Kennedy and the university in the 1970s. For Kennedy, dropping the issue of the Cincinnati research helped facilitate the passage of the first in a series of laws that would regulate federally funded medical research. For the university, forgetting—in this case, realized by disabling the formal qualities of memory spaces that enable public memory—prevented further damage to the reputations of the university and the doctors involved. Similarly, subsequent attempts at meaningful forgetting helped minimize the reputational fallout of the study again in the 1990s, which culminated in the creation of a memorial to the WBS's subjects that formally undercut the capacity for bioethical memory and witnessing.

University Recalcitrance and Meaningful Forgetting

The story of the Whole Body Radiation study went public on October 8, 1971, with an article that bluntly stated: "For the past 11 years, the Pentagon has had a contract with the University of Cincinnati to study the effect of atomic radiation on human beings. The prime purpose of the study, according to the contract, has been to 'understand better the influence of radiation on combat effectiveness of troops.'"[7] The article detailed how patients received the same radiation doses "that combat troops might expect to receive in an exchange of tactical nuclear weapons" and that "patients are not told that the Pentagon is funding their treatment or that the prime purpose of the research which they are part of is to understand the battlefield effects of radiation."[8] The *Washington Post* story had its genesis with Eugene Saenger and his willingness to share the details of his research with the media, until he started receiving negative coverage. Saenger first corresponded with Roger Rapoport from November 1970 through April 1971.[9] Rapoport included details shared by Saenger in his book *The Great American Bomb Machine*.[10] Saenger believed that excerpts of the book were then sent to the *New York Times* and

Washington Post.[11] As Saenger and others recount, Auerbach and O'Toole interviewed Saenger, DOD officials, and other sources during October 5–6 before publishing the article.[12]

The story had an immediate impact. Senator Kennedy announced the same day that he would investigate the Cincinnati research.[13] Other American newspapers picked up the *Washington Post* story, often adding more exaggerated or controversial headlines like the *Toledo Blade*'s "Pentagon Pact for Study of Radiation Revealed."[14] The story was also picked up by CBS and NBC and by media in England, France, Germany, and Israel.[15] On October 11, the University of Cincinnati held a press conference: Saenger along with Edward Gall, UC's vice president in charge of the Cincinnati General Hospital, and Clifford Grulee, the dean of the College of Medicine, defended the study.[16] Gall claimed to provide the only "accurate" and "rational" account of the study. He and Saenger emphasized that the patients were "fatally ill individuals" with no hope of a cure, but who would benefit from the "treatment" in terms of lengthening the time they survived with cancer. When asked to comment on the *Washington Post* story and the inaccuracies they claimed it had, both demurred. Gall claimed, "[I] have not read the story. I found it rather difficult to respond to slanted stories because I am not quite sure what is an allegation and what is an implication." Saenger said that responding "would be difficult to [do] . . . without going over this 'chapter and verse.'" Saenger claimed that the work he performed was treatment for disease and not research: "I do not believe we had guinea pigs in Cincinnati. Absolutely not. I think that these patients were carefully investigated; that there was a reason for treatment."

The press conference and its idealized—and inaccurate—vision of research were paradigmatic examples of physician responses to political and journalistic inquiry, mirroring the strategies David Rothman identified in the response of medical researchers to Walter Mondale and his proposals for research oversight.[17] Researchers' affiliation to their vision of themselves and medical research drove these initial responses. Yet, the press conference did not silence the public outcry or dampen congressional interest in the study.[18] This surprised the medical doctors. On

October 25, Gall wrote the UC public information office, "I would hope that we could delay any further features on the whole-body radiation until we know what the national climate will be. Do you think this would be feasible?"[19] In the essay "Ethics on Trial," which Saenger coauthored with Edward Silberstein, the two claim that they and the university were unable to answer the questions from the press and were "unprepared for the turmoil which lay ahead."[20] Much of this "turmoil" consisted of investigations by multiple groups.

One group that investigated the WBS study was the American College of Radiology (ACR). Their investigation was prompted by Senator Mike Gravel (D-AK), who sent the ACR a letter on November 10 listing a series of questions about the study and closing with the threat "to propose an amendment to the Defense Department's Appropriation Bill which would terminate Dr. Saenger's experimentation unless satisfactory answers have been provided to several questions."[21] The ACR, UC, and Saenger agreed to have a committee of physicians associated with the ACR investigate the study.[22] A three-man committee visited Cincinnati on December 16, and their report was transmitted to Gravel in the form of a letter from ACR president Robert McConnell on January 4, 1972. The letter opens by noting that Saenger's project "is validly conceived, stated, executed, controlled and followed up"; selection and enrollment of patients "conforms with good medical practice" and is "consistent with recommendations of the National Institutes of Health"; and it deserved Gravel's "support for its continuation."[23]

Yet, the review had severe limitations. It consisted of reading Saenger's publications and interviewing Saenger, his research team, and other university faculty and staff.[24] There was no contact with patients and no review of research documentation or patient records. The letter sidestepped the primary issues of concern for Gravel and others: The review assumed that the WBS study was clinical research of cancer rather than research on radiation exposures, and the "committee did not concern itself with the implications which have been raised concerning partial funding of the effort by the Department of Defense."[25] Whether the study was really clinical or not and the role of DOD funding were the key issues in the public controversy. The limits on the ACR investigation and the refusal to engage further when pressed reflect the philia of medical researchers generally and members of the ACR specifically. Medical professionals hoped to minimize outside meddling in their affairs. This was especially true for the insular ACR, whose critics noted its tendency to always protect its members.[26]

Another investigation was started by the University of Cincinnati in mid-November at the request of the university's new president, Warren Bennis.[27] The committee was organized by Clifford Grulee, the dean of the College of Medicine. This committee consisted of eleven members from the medical school and was led by Raymond Suskind, chair of the Environmental Health Center.[28] The names of the committee members were initially kept secret "in the interest of presenting a report as free from public pressure as possible."[29] The final 66-page report noted several flaws in data collection and other areas of the project, but it argued that if Saenger and colleagues made changes to the study protocol and found a new funding source, then the project could continue. Local newspaper accounts of the report framed it as an exoneration of Saenger and colleagues.[30] The public declarations again reflected the concord and affiliation of medical researchers.

Yet, internal deliberations at UC about the report and its implications were harsh. The tensions first began with the Suskind Committee itself. Some of the issues raised led to meetings lasting until midnight with no resolution in sight.[31] The poor quality of the WBS documentation and data was criticized during the committee's deliberations. In a January 12, 1972, memo from Raymond Suskind to committee members, he notes,

> According to Dr. Aron, it is not possible to develop any better information about palliation from the charts of the patients. . . . We also felt that suggesting a complete redoing of a Phase II study would have a very negative impact on both the patients and the research group itself. We felt that the best option was to use the very limited data in a constructive manner.[32]

Ironically, Dr. Bernard Aron, who had been involved with the WBS study in the mid-1960s, provided sharp criticism of Saenger's work within the private space of the committee's deliberations.[33] As the memo also noted, other members of the committee were equally critical within that space, although they tamped down that criticism when producing their final report. From late January through late April, Warren Bennis, Ed Gall, Raymond Suskind, provost Robert O'Neil, and committee member Vernon Stroud sent memos back and forth clarifying details of the report and debating what recommendations should be implemented, until Bennis decided on April 24 to accept the report's recommendations in their entirety.[34]

On January 25, the Junior Faculty Association (JFA), a group of untenured faculty at UC who were unaffiliated with the medical school, issued their own report on the WBS study, based on their reading of the reports Saenger and his colleagues made to the DOD. The report is sharply critical of Saenger and colleagues, and it challenges many of the assertions made by Saenger and university officials in defense of the study. The JFA report challenges claims that the WBS study was a clinical study of cancer treatment: "We have been unable to find any evidence of a planned, systematic, cancer study. It seems unlikely that the team would not have mentioned, somewhere in the 900 pages of the Department of Defense (D.O.D.) reports the fact that they were conducting the DOD project in conjunction with a specific cancer research study."[35] They challenge the claim that the study preexisted DOD funding ("There is no evidence in the DOD reports that any patients were irradiated before the beginning of the DOD project in February 1960"), and the claim that DOD concerns influenced patient treatment ("Consistently throughout the reports to the DOD the doctors make statements that indicate that the selection of patients and the radiation dose given them was at least partially tailored to the needs of the DOD project").[36] The report received limited media attention, but it was read into the *Congressional Record* by Senator Kennedy.[37]

Yet, these three investigations of the study pale in comparison to the time and attention given to it by Senator Edward M. Kennedy

and his staff. The day the *Washington Post* story appeared, one of Senator Kennedy's staff, Ellis Mottur, informed Kennedy of the story and
began an investigation of the study.[38] Kennedy, along with Senator
Walter Mondale (D-MN) had been trying to pass legislation that would
regulate medical research.[39] They believed that hearings on abuses of
medical research would facilitate the legislation's passage. Initially,
Kennedy and his staff tried to move rapidly and incorporate testimony
about the WBS research into hearings in early November, but there
is no indication in the *Congressional Record* or the extant archives on the
study that this happened.[40] Eventually two Senate staffers—Ellis Mottur
and Phillip Capur—visited Cincinnati on December 6, where they met
with a number of individuals including Eugene Saenger, Edward Silberstein, and Edward Gall. During the visit, the two staffers requested
that the research team provide access to the surviving patients in order
for them to be interviewed about the experience of consenting to the
study. Saenger and Silberstein separately wrote memos detailing their
encounters with Mottur and Capur. They are clear about the defensive,
hostile, and sometimes legalistic nature of their answers. Silberstein
notes he told the two staffers that it was "a political issue here rather
than our study."[41] Saenger is even more vocal, especially on the issue of
interviews:

> This is a personal impression of mine but there is no question in my
> mind that these men would dearly love to get directly at the patients
> and exploit them in any way possible. . . . It seemed reasonably clear
> that the issues concerning our research were not nearly as important in
> their minds as in using this issue to get at the advisability of Department
> of Defense funding for this project. If they could hobble the D.O.D.
> in this research they could hobble the D.O.D. in all other biomedical
> research whenever they would chose to do so.[42]

The interviews, and the possibility of later testimony before Congress,
were key. Without people willing to describe their experiences and to
embody the arguments about medicine's ethical failings, proposals to

regulate medical research would have a difficult time becoming law.[43] Saenger's and Silberstein's suspicions reflect this reality, but distort it into a personal and "political" attack on them that had more to do with Congress than with research. The need to preserve research practice as it existed at that time and the related identity of medical researchers played a substantial role in Saenger's and Silberstein's actions.

These suspicions also led to Saenger's campaign over the next two months to prevent Senator Kennedy and his staff from having contact with the surviving research subjects, a campaign that the university itself joined. A handwritten note from Edward Silberstein to Edward Gall, written on behalf of the research team, notes, "It is the unanimous opinion of the three of us as well as the project director, Dr. E.L. Saenger, that such an *inquisition* could only be harmful to these women psychologically and, hence, medically. . . . We four thus feel it is in the best interest of our patients to protect them from the stresses and possible tragic consequences of this investigation."[44] Saenger himself wrote letters to Gall and Charles Bennett, chair of the radiology department, on several occasions, urging them to refuse Kennedy and Mottur's requests for interviews: In a December 17 letter to Bennett, he warned, "With a few adroitly phrased questions, it would be comparatively easy to convey an impression to the public that these patients had been grievously exploited especially using techniques of 'leading the witness.'"[45]

On December 22, 1971, Edward Gall wrote to Senator Kennedy to inform him that they would not make subjects in the study available for interviews:

> I have discussed this request with both medical and legal authorities and have made the decision that I cannot comply with your request. Primarily this is deemed ill-advised and not in the best medical interests of the patients. Moreover legal counsel have informed me that I have no authority to reveal the identity of a patient under the existing circumstances. This would constitute a violation of Ohio law relating to privilege [*sic*] communication between physician and patient. It would, in addition, constitute a breach of a patient's right to privacy.[46]

It is not clear who Gall consulted on this besides Saenger, Silberstein, and possibly Barrett, especially since the legal arguments Gall presented in his letter to the senator were baseless. This is clear in a letter from UC's general counsel to Warren Bennis: "It is possible that you are accountable to the Congressional Committee for the University's refusal to release to a Congressional Committee the names of the patients in the total body radiation program."[47] The letter notes that congressional committees have the right to any information within their legislative mandate, unless limited explicitly by the Constitution or a finding by a federal court, and that Ohio's laws on patient-physician privilege are not involved in the case. The letter closes with the observation that "the only justification advanced for withholding the names which is relevant at the present stage is that subjecting the patients to a decision to submit to an interview by the Committee's staff would substantially impair the health of the patients."[48] Kennedy and his staff knew this also, as is clear in a *Cincinnati Enquirer* article: "But Mottur said preliminary checks with Library of Congress legal experts 'Make it seen [*sic*] unlikely that what he [Gall] said about Ohio law will prove to be the case. We're not asking for any information about the patients, but just want them to have the free right to talk to us.'"[49]

The fight over access to the research subjects took an odd turn after Kennedy and his staff discovered that subjects were interviewed by National Educational Television in September 1971 for a documentary on the research.[50] These interviews had been arranged by Eugene Saenger and Edward Silberstein. The UC administration had been unaware of these interviews until informed by Senator Kennedy that they existed.[51] Saenger described his failure to tell anyone as a "personal error" resulting from "being naïve," and he concludes, "In the absence of any impropriety [on my part] I will continue to regard this matter as one of lack of recall and not as a failure of good faith or intent."[52] The next day, he wrote a letter to Gall and Barrett encouraging them to shift their answers to Kennedy: He urged them to tell Kennedy that the university refused to grant interviews now because of a "change in our attitude following the *Washington Post* article of October 8" but that "we should rethink a flat out refusal for any type of interview . . . in this way we do not appear so rigid."[53] This strategy was successfully pitched to Cincinnati's local newspapers, who depicted UC as operating in good faith and as seriously considering Kennedy's request.[54] Gall also used that framing in his response to Kennedy on January 19.[55] While they were resisting Kennedy's demands, the university also solicited opinions from physician-researchers across the country as to the inadvisability of allowing the patients to be interviewed, and queried the surviving patients about their willingness to be interviewed.[56]

The debate between Kennedy and UC about the right to interview patients overlapped with the ACR, Suskind, and JFA reports. Media attention was focused on this issue. Kennedy, looking to address an issue he prioritized, saw this situation as one likely to facilitate the regulation of medical research. Yet, by the end of April, the university turned down additional funding from the Defense Department, Kennedy dropped his request for patient interviews, and media attention rapidly dwindled away. By the end of the year, the case of Cincinnati's total body radiation study had been all but forgotten by the public.

FORGETTING THE STUDY

Between March and late April, stories about the Cincinnati WBS study began to circulate with less frequency as Kennedy and his staff stopped trying to get access to patients and the Suskind Committee's investigation was wound down. After the university refused any further funding from the DOD, there was almost no further discussion of the Cincinnati WBS study until August, when brief mention of it was made during the passage of legislation placing informed consent requirements on research funded by the Department of Defense.[57] According to Martha Stephens, further discussion was suppressed through backroom dealings between the University of Cincinnati, Ohio governor John Gilligan, and Senator Kennedy:

The school stepped up its efforts with their political friends to get them
off what was now a very sharp hook. . . . In time, Bennis met with Kennedy and with Kennedy's fellow liberal and friend, Ohio governor John
Gilligan, and the three of them made a pact: Kennedy would agree to
no interviews with patients and no congressional investigation into the
basement chambers, in exchange for the halting of the project by UC,
or at least the refusal of any further funds from the DOD.[58]

Stephens turned to an article in UC's student newspaper, the *News Record,* as the source for their claim, but the article only says that Bennis,
Gilligan, Kennedy, and Charles Bennett had met. It quotes Bennis: "I
don't think the meeting had any more specific conclusions."[59] Stephens
might have been swayed to this view of events by several factors. First,
there are no details about the meeting in the archival material at the University of Cincinnati or the ACHRE archives.[60] Second, in subsequent
conversations in March and April about the implications of the Suskind
report, Bennis does not provide any indication as to his thinking or his
plans regarding the recommendations in the report. This absence can be
mobilized in a narrative of a backroom deal that overrode other considerations at the university level.

Archival material from the papers of Senator Robert Taft Jr. (R-
OH), which was unavailable to Stephens, and retrospective accounts
from John Gilligan and former Kennedy staffers undermine the conspiracy version of the study's end. On February 24—immediately after
the meeting—Kennedy wrote Gilligan. He thanked him for arranging
the meeting, and he appreciated the "kind offer to help facilitate the
Health Subcommittee inquiry into the University of Cincinnati's Radiation Project. Your assurance of making the necessary arrangements for
Subcommittee communication with the patients or their families should
prove most helpful."[61] The next day Charles Barrett talked with Taft by
phone about the meeting. According to Taft's handwritten notes, Barrett
said that Kennedy and Bennis "left on basis of decision after GAO and
review of report of Medical School."[62] In 1994, when the story became
public again, John Gilligan told news reporters that "he offered to act as

an 'intermediary' between investigators from Kennedy's committee and UC officials but the investigation was dropped just as he and his staff were getting involved."[63] In other words, no decision had been made about the investigation at the February 24 meeting. Barrett indicated that a decision would await receiving both a report from the General Accounting Office about the contracts between UC and the DOD and Kennedy's review of the Medical School report. Kennedy's own words at the time indicate that he still intended to move forward with seeking interviews of the patients.

Instead of conspiracy, three factors led to Kennedy's decision to drop the investigation. First, Saenger and his colleagues, especially Edward Silberstein, made it difficult—if not impossible—for Kennedy to secure the cooperation of the research subjects. On January 18, Silberstein sent a letter to each of the participants with a return envelope. The message read:

> A member of the United States Senate wants to send a person to talk with you about your sickness and treatment. They want me to give them your name and tell them where you live, but I have refused to give them this information without your O.K.
>
> Do you want me to give them your name?[64]

Silberstein frames the congressional request as a gross violation of the individual's privacy: the unnamed senator wants to know about "*your* sickness and treatment" and wants to know the person's name and address. Silberstein appears to be a defender of their privacy, refusing to provide the information without the patient's agreement. This position reflects the mid-twentieth-century beliefs about the doctor-patient relationship as the moral foundation of medicine and a relationship that was entirely private.[65] Such wording also deflects attention away from accusations of wrongdoing on the part of Silberstein and Saenger: it is about the person's "sickness," not the accusation that the patient was used for medical experimentation. In doing this, Silberstein made interviews appear like a gross imposition by an unnamed senator on the patients, thus making it unlikely that the subject would be willing to talk.[66] These documents were sent to Ellis Mottur, along with the letters from the outside consultants arguing against the interviews in early February.[67]

Second, in addition to undercutting the ability to interview patients, Saenger and colleagues worked with their political contacts to stall or stop Kennedy's investigation. Their primary ally in this effort was the then-freshman senator Robert Taft Jr.[68] According to Saenger's personal notes, he and Taft had close ties.[69] Taft became an ardent defender of the university and Saenger. According to Ellis Mottur, "Taft went bonkers on this thing."[70] Yet, Taft's initial forays were much quieter than Mottur recalled, or possibly knew. Taft had been in contact with physicians at the University of Cincinnati shortly after the WBS story received national attention in October. According to his files, Taft had created a press release defending the university from the allegations in the *Washington Post* story and the concerns raised by Kennedy, but UC's Charles Barrett encouraged Taft to not make a statement while the university sought opinions from "indisputable experts" to aid its defense.[71] Taft held his tongue for the next two months, quietly querying the DOD about the study and keeping tabs on the Senate Subcommittee on Health's investigation.[72]

Taft eventually felt he needed to speak out, despite requests from UC that he wait until the university had received the expert reviews and advice it supposedly had been soliciting.[73] On December 15, Taft took to the Senate floor on a day when Kennedy was absent from Washington to denounce him and his investigation. Taft demanded that hearings by the Senate Subcommittee on Health be scheduled immediately to answer the charges Taft felt Kennedy had made against UC's WBS program: "I do not believe that charges as serious as these should be simply made and forgotten. . . . When a leading university medical center is accused of running little more than a death camp for cancer patients, I believe that the public has a legitimate interest in a full and complete inquiry."[74] He complained, "This investigation was launched in Cincinnati without my knowledge, without any resolution adopted by the Health subcommittee . . . [and] more importantly, I question the propriety of issuing public statements on the basis of a field trip by majority staffers."[75]

Taft's claim that Kennedy was accusing the University of Cincinnati of operating a "death camp" on the basis of a staffer's "field trip" became fodder for numerous Ohio newspapers.[76] Taft's interest was a mixed blessing for the UC doctors. An undated memo attached to a draft of Taft's December 15 statement included a message from UC's Barrett, saying the statement was "too long, too involved and challenging Kennedy to open the conflict further," and encouraged Taft to wait until they had received the expert reviews of the program.[77] In fact, a December 17 *Cincinnati Enquirer* article quoted Ellis Mottur: "We will probably have public hearings now that Sen. (Robert) Taft (Jr.) (R-Ohio) has emphasized that he wants them."[78] The university had resisted being drawn into Senate hearings on the issue, but their own ally undercut their desires with his own demands for hearings where he could excoriate Kennedy's statements on Cincinnati.

Yet, Taft's attacks would eventually contribute to Kennedy dropping the idea of hearings and interviews with research subjects. According to Taft's archives, every time he received a statement, news article, or any other item where Kennedy or his staff mentioned the Cincinnati WBS study, Taft would write a letter, press release, or speech denouncing Kennedy and defending Saenger and colleagues. After Kennedy wrote Taft to correct inaccuracies from his December 15 speech, Taft wrote Kennedy and declared, "I regret any inaccuracies in my earlier letter. Perhaps they are not surprising in view of the fact that, as far as I know, no committee authorization has taken place and up until the last week or so neither minority staff nor my staff were being apprised of any actions being taken by majority staff members."[79] Taft accused Kennedy of acting inappropriately in investigating the Cincinnati experiments without subcommittee authorization, although Kennedy as subcommittee chair did not require approval from the committee, a fact known to Taft even as he leveled the accusation.[80] Nonetheless, Taft continued accusing Kennedy of impropriety through January 1972.[81]

Finally, at some point in early 1972, Kennedy decided to let the issue of the Cincinnati study drop. According to Mottur, "Kennedy felt if we got into this battle with Taft it would divert attention from the really constructive purposes we were trying to achieve."[82] Kennedy did inadvertently mention the study one more time in July 1972 while asking for support from the Health Subcommittee for an amendment to DOD appropriations that would place requirements for informed consent on DOD-funded research.[83] Ellis Mottur called Taft's staff to apologize for the reference, and told them "Kennedy will not mention Cincinnati during the debate on the amendment."[84]

Overall, pressure from Senator Taft (encouraged by Saenger and other UC doctors) and Silberstein's manipulation of research subjects led to Kennedy's investigation being dropped. UC and Saenger kept their reputations, even as the practices on which medical research's identity were based eroded. Kennedy succeeded later in 1972 in mandating informed consent for participants in DOD-funded research. The parties in this debate allowed the study to drop from public consciousness. They strategically forgot it because doing so allowed them to achieve their desired goals—maintained reputation for some, and research regulation for others—by other means. In doing so, they undermined the early circulation of the story needed to enable its development into bioethical public memory.

IMPEDING FURTHER CIRCULATION OF THE STORY

After the investigations concluded and the funding for the study stopped, faculty at UC worked to maintain the meaningful forgetting accomplished in 1972 and prevent the study from being recalled and re-membered, as is illustrated by events in 1974 and 1975. In 1974, a visiting professor from Barnard College, Bradford Gray, would write Raymond Suskind, who chaired the university's review committee, to ask him for a copy of the report.[85] Suskind responded, "I shall be happy to send you a copy of the report if you can give me some idea as to what kind of study you are engaged in and how the report relates to your work."[86] Gray "was a bit taken back" by Suskind's request, although he then charitably noted that "given the sensitivity of the issues involved . . . your caution is not so surprising."[87] Gray then reassures Suskind that he hopes to offer "a serious discussion and sociological analysis" and that he primarily wants the report out of "a strong preference for examining all available information on the subject."[88] Gray's emphasis on his serious sociological analysis—along with the indication that Gray only asked for the report out of a desire for thoroughness—mollified Suskind, who sent the report, minus its appendices, with a note that he initially balked as "a matter of discretion."[89] Gray then asked for the appendices.[90] He received them, along with the request that he inform Suskind "how, if at all, some of this material will be used in your study."[91] Suskind restricted access to the report until he was sufficiently assured that the reasons were appropriately academic, but even then, he wanted to keep close tabs on whether it would circulate in that smaller, rarefied setting.

The desire to suppress the circulation of the story became even more apparent the next year. While Suskind wanted to control how information about the WBS study and its aftermath circulated, Eugene Saenger and Edward Silberstein, the study's primary investigators, wanted to voice their outrage at the closure of the WBS study. Their essay "Ethics on Trial: Medical, Congressional, and Journalistic" presents the events of 1971–1972 as an unjustified persecution of the two men by ignorant politicians and journalists, abetted by the university's public relations incompetence and the university president's cowardice.[92] The essay's persecution narrative, according to Martha Stephens, shows "Saenger and Silberstein still smarting and suffering under the loss of the whole body project and almost incredulous that with the nearly uniform medical support for their work in Cincinnati and around the country things could have come to so sorry a conclusion."[93] After they completed it, the two sent the draft to a number of UC faculty and administrators, as well as individuals outside of the university who had been involved with the controversy. They tell the recipients, "We would appreciate your critical comments as to whether this account of our experience adds to the understanding of circumstances concerning human research. . . . do you feel this account is accurate? Please make comments concerning the manuscript and its possible scientific value."[94]

Some recipients sympathized. "Your letter . . . makes me realize for the first time what a nightmare you have lived with," said William Beierwaltes.[95] Others offered tepid endorsement of it: Charles Barrett briefly told the two "fine article—well done," while McConnell from the ACR noted, "I feel it represents a reasonably accurate summary of your experiences and events that have transpired."[96] Most who received the essay explicitly encouraged the two to drop the issue.[97] Beierwaltes counsels, "It sounds as though the investigational problems and criticisms have cooled and that you now have more time to devote to more constructive work. . . . I do not believe the publication would serve any constructive purpose."[98] In response to an earlier draft, Gall advised, "Frankly, although a grievous experience, it has gone through the sluice gate and is well down stream. My own reaction is to avoid chasing after it to bring it back into the fore."[99] ACR's Otha Linton told the two, "My overall subjective response would be some reluctance to have you publish it as it exists now. I think it would create an additional furor in Washington at a time when this matter and the broader matter of 'human experimentation' is not currently active."[100]

Recipients of Silberstein and Saenger's narrative are sympathetic to the two but raise concerns about publishing it. To circulate the narrative—to remind people of what happened at UC—would raise the issue of human subjects research at a time when it had faded from public attention. In other words, those—like Gall and Linton—who were closely associated with the events in 1971 and 1972 persuaded Saenger and Silberstein to drop the issue. Ultimately, Silberstein and Saenger did set aside the essay, and the story of the whole body radiation study was generally forgotten. In fact, even attempts to raise the issue of radiation research generally—attempts like the 1986 Markey Committee report *American Nuclear Guinea Pigs: Three Decades of Radiation Experiments on U.S. Citizens*—are largely ignored.[101] These acts of forgetting work to the benefit of Saenger and his colleagues, whose reputations remain intact, and to the university, which does not find itself associated with problematic research and medicine gone wrong in the way that the Jewish Chronic Disease Hospital, the Willowbrook School, and others were.

The Story Resurfaces

Efforts to stop the investigation of Saenger's research in 1972 and subsequently to contain or suppress further circulation of the story succeeded for more than twenty years, but Saenger's research received renewed attention in 1993 when energy secretary Hazel O'Leary announced that the federal government had supported research that exposed people to radiation without their knowledge.[102] The university tried to downplay the story, as they had done in the 1970s: they issued a statement "calling the reports on the study 'old news.'"[103] This time, when local media were confronted with the story, they did not support the university and Saenger as they had in the 1970s. Saenger had retired in 1987. This time, there was no flurry of memos from Saenger to the president of the university, dean of the medical school, and others dictating, or attempting to dictate, the university's responses to events. Saenger's political benefactor, Robert Taft Jr., had died in December 1993, leaving him without someone to forestall further investigation by the federal government. And there were many investigations. Yet, Saenger, the university, and their defenders were able to stymie the investigations and subsequent attempts to memorialize those who died in the study. We can see this when we examine the national investigation, embodied in the ACHRE final report, and then the memorial for victims created as part of the outcome of the lawsuit against the university.

THE ACHRE REPORT

O'Leary's revelation of federal support for radiation experiments on Americans prompted President Bill Clinton to form the Advisory Committee on Human Radiation Experiments (ACHRE).[104] The committee's mission was ambitious and daunting. ACHRE spent two years trying to account for the thousands of experiments conducted by the federal government in the mid-twentieth century involving the study of radiation. They also assessed the practices of biomedical research in the mid-1990s to see what ethical lapses might still occur. They developed a framework for making retrospective moral judgments, and they eventually offered a series of recommendations to the president and Congress on how to respond to past studies and how to prevent future abuses.[105] Among the thousands of Cold War–era experiments identified, the Cincinnati WBS study was selected for closer examination.[106] Yet, even as the case was identified as an important one, the radiologists on the committee were making public statements denying that Saenger's work was ethically suspect or that it should even be viewed as military research.[107] In doing so, the radiologists undercut a key element of bioethical public memory: the capacity of memory's witnesses to offer, or to facilitate, a judgment about injustice and tragedy, responsibility and absolution. Without responsibility or the ability to contemplate where responsibility for past injustice lies, the capacity of bioethical memory's audiences to act as witnesses is hampered, if not undone.

ACHRE's ethical judgment of radiation experiments is bifurcated. In the substantive chapter describing the Cincinnati study, the judgments made are explicit, definitive, and harsh:

> In the case of the Cincinnati experiments, the impact of the research protocol on the care of the patient-subjects cannot be construed as beneficial to the patients. . . . To the extent that this deviated from standard of care, and caused unnecessary suffering and discomfort, it was morally unconscionable; to the extent that the standard of care in this area is uncertain, it is morally questionable. As troubling as this is, far more troubling is the evidence, including the testimony of the principal investigator, that TBI [Total Body Irradiation] might not have even been employed, or once employed continued, in the absence of the government's funding and research requirements.[108]

Yet, despite this condemnation—and equally strong statements on other experiments ACHRE studied in depth—the committee's overall conclusions and recommendations are tepid. The committee crafted narrow criteria for financial and medical compensation, arguing that an apology was an appropriate remedy for many of the cases studied. Yet even the apology was viewed as too much by some members of the committee. They feared that they might apologize to too many people and that identifying who deserved an apology was too daunting a task.[109] Compensation was identified as an appropriate response to individuals who underwent WBS or their families, if it was "determined that WBS was considered at the time to be a controversial treatment."[110] After offering a strong condemnation of the Cincinnati WBS case, the report's conclusion distances itself from that condemnation.

The failure to close the report with stronger condemnations of radiation studies generally and WBS studies specifically was the result of an epistemological filibuster by some committee members. According to Marcus Paroske, an epistemological filibuster is the strategic use of "uncertainty over how thoroughly to deliberate as a means to preclude the resolution of that issue in government action."[111] Allan Buchanan noted that some members objected from the outset to making retrospective ethical judgments, and after grudgingly agreeing to a framework for judgment, they challenged the standards for evidence and then the strength of the evidence.[112] By enacting this filibuster, some committee members with affiliations or sympathies to radiology and to Saenger undercut the possibility for judgment. In doing so, their actions, as enshrined in the ACHRE report, impeded the central tasks of bioethical memory—witnessing and judgment—thus contributing to the inability of the public to remember radiation experiments and the WBS.

CINCINNATI MEMORIAL

While deliberations and investigations were taking place in Washington, the families of Cincinnati WBS subjects filed a federal lawsuit.[113] The families sued the University of Cincinnati, the City of Cincinnati, Cincinnati Children's Hospital Medical Center, the United States government, and eleven individual doctors, including Eugene Saenger and Edward Silberstein, for a range of civil rights violations, including "the right of access to the courts, the right to privacy, to bodily integrity, and to make decisions about their own bodies."[114] Ultimately, the case was settled out of court.[115] In addition to remuneration for families of the research's subjects, the settlement included a requirement for a plaque "to honor those who were involved in the Pentagon-funded research and died."[116] On its face, the plaque might indicate a collective agreement that the university assumes a moral responsibility for the WBS study and a responsibility for remembering the study and those it harmed. Yet, the plaque's history, content, and placement are an attempt at *mnemonicide,* the "erasure of memory as it occurs at a specific historical moment."[117] While such attempts at forgetting might not be absolutely success-ful—the historical record about the study persists—they undermine the symbolic and material supports necessary to allow any specific historical content to become public memory.

The legal wrangling over the plaque during the settlement illustrates how the university divorced itself from the responsibility for the study and for enabling public memory of it. The initial settlement proposed that "the defendant University of Cincinnati shall accept a plaque . . . and place such plaque in a suitable location on the campus of the University of Cincinnati."[118] The initial proposal indicated the university would place a 12 × 25 inch plaque in an undetermined location. The plaque would have the title "In Memoriam," followed by the initials of those who died in the experiment, with the statement "presented by their families" appearing below the initials.[119] Judge Beckwith rejected the original settlement proposal in part because of the proposal for the plaque, arguing:

> The settlement agreement does not indicate where the plaque will be placed. Perhaps more significantly, the agreement does not indicate who will determine which location is suitable for the placement of the plaque. . . . The Court is not persuaded, however, that those class mem-bers value the mere acceptance of the plaque, rather than its placement in a location that is suitable from their perspective.[120]

As the judge noted, there were a series of defects with the proposed me-morial. First, the lack of a clear location cut at one of the key qualities

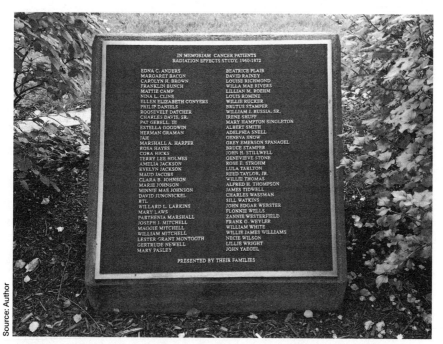

Figure 6. The Cincinnati Whole Body Radiation study memorial plaque includes the names of most subjects of the study and the dates the study ran. The text emphasizes that the plaque was presented by their families and does not mention the lawsuit mandating its placement.

of memorials—place. Place is key to the ability of memorials and the memories they articulate to be noticed and to circulate. Second, by only including the subjects' initials, the plaque worked to minimize, if not outright eliminate, the traces of the subjects and their names. Third, by ending with "presented by their families," the proposed plaque accurately reflected that the plaque was demanded by the families, but it distances the university from the memorial and the responsibility for remembering the study. A revised proposal that included a larger plaque with the full names of seventy of the WBS subjects and an established location at University Hospital met with Beckwith's approval.[121]

The content of the plaque also undercut its ability to foster public memory of the study. In fact, the plaque better reflects the concerns of researchers and the university who were afraid "the plaque would be misinterpreted as an admission of guilt," rather than the concerns of the families.[122] The plaque opens with the dedication "In Memoriam Cancer Patients/Radiation Effects Study, 1960–1972." It then lists the names of seventy individuals who had been in the study, and then closes with the statement "presented by their families" (see figure 6). Like the proposed plaque, the actual plaque keeps the language of "presented by their families," obscuring responsibility for remembering the study. Unlike the initial proposal, the plaque names the individuals, recognizes they were cancer patients, and links them to the WBS study. Yet, the plaque sidesteps the details of what the "radiation effects study" was, what it did, and how or why these cancer patients were involved. The plaque minimizes details about the study and the degree to which the study is responsible for the subject's deaths, ultimately effacing any indications of guilt. This differs from the "minimal remembrance" enabled by the Willowbrook monuments because memory of the Cincinnati studies did not—and do not—circulate as widely as the details of the Willowbrook State School and the conditions that existed there.

Finally, and most troubling, the successive locations of the plaque undermine the power of place, which is essential to memorializing. A *Cincinnati Enquirer* article provides an evocative, melancholic description of the plaque's initial location in 1999:

> Nestled in an old corner of the University Hospital grounds stands a sad little courtyard with a single tree, three park benches, and two picnic tables that once was called a "therapeutic garden."
>
> Patients haven't used this place in years. An oval asphalt walkway is crumbled and broken. The sign that calls this spot a garden is rusted and broken in half. There isn't a flower to be seen.
>
> These days, employees use the courtyard as a place to catch a smoke or sometimes eat their lunch.[123]

Another article published the same day in the *Enquirer* notes, "The plaque is in a courtyard near Burnet and Elland avenues on the University of

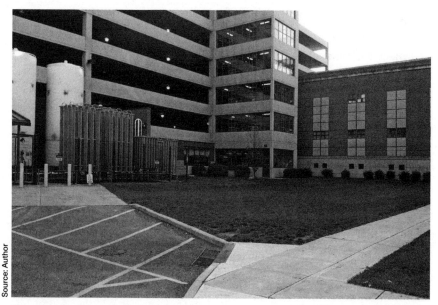

Source: Author

Figure 7. The Cincinnati WBS memorial is located at the back of a parking garage. None of the walkways in the area, with the exception of the garage exit, passes near the memorial.

Cincinnati campus. The courtyard, between Pavilions H and J, includes ventilation units and a tree."[124]

The location of the plaque is *quasi-public*. Its poor condition and the uses to which it is put work to erase the memories it ostensibly creates on two levels. First, the location itself is rarely used by anyone. According to the news reports, only hospital employees used the space for lunch and to smoke; patients and the general public would not generally use the space or move through it. Place is key to a memorial's capacity to foster memory, and this location undercuts that capacity. In addition to issues of access, the condition of the location itself sends a message that nothing of value exists in the space. The "therapeutic garden" is in disrepair, with rusted signage and broken pathways, indicating that any value the space had for visitors or the public is long past. The anemic trees and the large ventilation units, along with the disrepair, mark the space as a neglected one that no longer has value for the public or the community as public space. The therapeutic garden is now only useful as a quasi-public space, repurposed as the location for hospital infrastructure and as a place for employees to eat and smoke.

In 2001, the nearby Pavilion J that bounded one half of the therapeutic garden was demolished to make way for a parking garage.[125] The plaque was moved to another "nearby courtyard . . . near an outdoor smoking area" while the building of the parking garage was completed.[126] Then, the plaque was moved back into the open space next to the parking garage, where the reorganization of the physical space and placement of the memorial plaque continued to undermine the memory work of the plaque. Again, the renovated location is only quasi-public. The space is located at the back of several buildings and a parking garage (figure 7). To access it from the street, rather than these structures, one must walk up a driveway, and past a parking lot and an emergency generator for the hospital, until one encounters a grassy area with a tree and a few bushes. There is no signage or other markers indicating that anything of value exists here. There is no direct path from the parking lot area to the memorial plaque. The only sidewalk that ends at the parking lot does not go near the memorial plaque. In addition to its general placement, the orientation of the plaque in this space helps undercut work to remember the study: specifically, the plaque faces toward the parking garage and not the open green space behind it (figure 8).

From 2010 through 2016, the plaque and its plinth were also obscured by shrubbery that had grown and hidden them. The shrubbery also obscures the view of the plaque from the parking garage: A short concrete path goes from the back exit of the parking garage to an entrance to the hospital. While this goes past the low-lying plaque, the shrubbery had obscured it (figure 9). The plaque and its current location work to forget the Cincinnati WBS study. Its location undermines the ability for minimal recognition provided by the plaque for the subjects of the study. Siting the plaque in a neglected, quasi-public space with the only path to the monument going from the back exit of a parking garage to an adjacent building results in minimal foot traffic past the memorial. Combined with the fact that the plaque faces the garage and is obscured

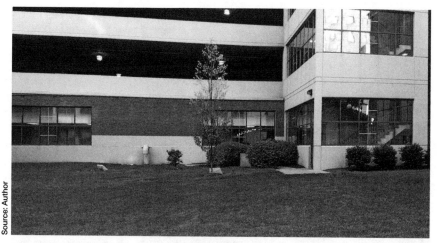

Source: Author

Figure 8. In this photograph from October 2012, the memorial is overgrown by the surrounding shrubs.

by shrubbery, it is clear that its location and content are mnemonicidal, working to suppress circulation of memories of the WBS study.

The attempt at mnemonicide had been largely successful. In 2008, I discussed the study with undergraduate students in a rhetoric of science course. Almost all of the students were Cincinnati natives—and a number of them lived in the same communities where the subjects' surviving families lived—but none of them knew about the study. They were shocked that something like this had ever happened. Two years later, I discovered that a colleague in the anthropology department who teaches about health and medicine sends his graduate and undergraduate students to the medical campus every year to look for the memorial plaque. He told me then that they always struggle and often fail to find the plaque without his help, and as late as 2016, they were still having difficulty finding it.[127]

Yet attempts at forgetting—the undermining of the material and symbolic matrix that allows memory to become public—are never *absolutely* successful. As long as the memory contents exist in public, in individual memory, or in historical archives, the work of forgetting can be undone.

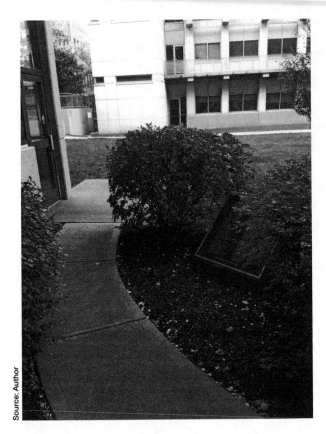

Source: Author

Figure 9. Pathway
from parking garage
into next building,
with Cincinnati
WBS memorial
plaque obscured
by bushes, October
2012.

In June 2017, the blog *Fear and Loathing in Bioethics* posted a story about
the WBS memorial. It detailed the physical location of the plaque and
its problems, and it also included images showing how the shrubbery
around the plaque had engulfed and completely obscured it.[128] The blog
post renewed public attention to the study, undoing the obscurity and
forgetfulness engendered over the years since the plaque was placed in
a quasi-public space. A local news channel ran a story on the memorial's condition.[129] The attention led the university to relandscape the area
and install low-lying plants that would not obscure the plaque. Yet, in
responding to the story, the university defers responsibility for maintaining the memorial and downplays the value of memorials. The press release notes, "When notified that the memorial had been unintentionally

covered by overgrown landscaping, the issue was addressed with new landscaping within hours to prevent this from occurring again."[130] While highlighting their actions to make the memorial visible, the press release defers responsibility for proactively maintaining the memorial, sidestepping the lack of active maintenance and the choice to landscape the area with plants that would inevitably obscure the memorial if the space were not maintained.

The press release also notes that the university and society as a whole have learned "a great deal" since the WBS study "on the ethical responsibilities of informed participation in research":

> Our role is not only to do the research to advance healthcare, but to protect the patients involved in that research. As such, memorials are not enough. Our efforts are to never let this happen again, and to let this legacy be the real memorial to the patients. This is why community advocates often serve on our Institutional Review Boards to help monitor the research and the process of informed consent.[131]

The statement downplays the importance of public memory and memorials: action, not memory, is what is important. Yet, the actions they describe—including community advocates on IRBs—is mandated by law and is not a free choice by the university to meet ethical obligations. Ultimately, the changes to the landscaping do very little to alter how the material and spatial arrangement of the plaque works to foster forgetting: the memorial is still hard to find and access, and the plaque still faces away from any public traffic.

Conclusion

Many people are familiar with the Tuskegee Study of Untreated Syphilis. Some are aware of the Willowbrook Hepatitis Study. But very few people remember the Cincinnati Whole Body Radiation Study. While it is described in histories of research ethics and received two book-length historical and ethical treatments, public remembrance has been minimal and arguably nonexistent. The *public availability of discourse* on the study does not equal *public discourse* about the study, much less public memory. Just because discourse was available, it did not become a focus of collective concern and judgment. Public memory, including bioethical public memory, requires either instantiation in discourses that are actively circulated over long periods of time or instantiation in places through which people circulate. They require a set of symbolic and material supports—alongside sufficient details of the events—to prompt individual recollection of the shared narratives constituting public memory.

Such qualities do not exist in the case of the Cincinnati radiation studies. This is a result of at least two acts of forgetting. The first is the deliberate, meaningful forgetting of the story in the early 1970s. Senator Ted Kennedy wanted to create federal regulations of research that would require informed consent. Resistance from the university and Senator Robert Taft Jr. made investigations of the Cincinnati research an impractical vehicle for achieving that goal. Thus, Kennedy dropped the case in order to pursue other avenues toward research regulation and requiring informed consent. When the WBS study became news again in the 1990s, the university accepted a lawsuit settlement wherein a memorial would be created, but the university was given such latitude with the creation of the memorial that it actually becomes a form of *forgetfulness,* working to suppress the public's ability to remember the study. It is an act of mnemonicide for the sake of creating a past unblemished by accusations of research misconduct.

The desire to hide troubling and unsightly details of the past is both unsurprising and a reflection of the power of philia. There was—and is—resistance to claims that research in the 1960s and 1970s was unethical from medical researchers. Their communal identity, especially the concord or *homonoia* about what research was and how to conduct it, was threatened by public exposure and demands that politicians, journalists, and research participants themselves have a say in clinical and research practice. What is unique here are the ways that the Cincinnati WBS study has been forgotten: first strategically to realize regulation of DOD-funded research, and second to outright suppress a specific memory that blemishes a storied reputation. UC and the affiliated hospitals are the birthplace of the first oral polio vaccine and the first antihistamine, Benadryl, among other accomplishments. The WBS study is a dark mark on this history. The fact that the university created a memorial that works to undercut the qualities necessary to facilitate public memory is a dubious, but remarkable, achievement.

While families of the WBS subjects and their advocates might be equally outraged by both moments of forgetting, the two should not be treated as functionally equivalent, as occurs in the most thorough account of the study by Martha Stephens. Pursuing hearings of the Cincinnati WBS study in 1971 was a means to the end of research regulation; Kennedy deciding to drop the issue and strategically allowing its memory to fade and be forgotten was a different means to the same end. Forgetting the harms done to past individuals unfortunately became part of the legislative calculus for preventing further harms in the present and the future. While we might wish things were otherwise, the dynamics of power and senatorial prerogatives—combined with the interference of the researchers—allowed Robert Taft Jr. to stymie the attempts of Kennedy and his staff to investigate the study.

The outcome in the 1990s is more ethically troubling. The university agreed to individual compensation for the families of the WBS subjects, and they agreed to "injunctive relief" in the form of the memorial plaque and the promise to abide by conventions for human subjects research and informed consent. This time, the families did receive consideration and compensation, but the promise to adhere to conventions for research was a pointless one: The university was already bound to adhere to human subjects requirements by federal regulations that applied to any university receiving federal research funds. Basically, the university agreed to adhere to the laws that they were already required to obey. Furthermore, the settlement of the lawsuit allowed the university to control how the study was memorialized, and they decided to craft a plaque whose content and location worked to suppress the circulation of narratives about the WBS study.

Conclusion

————•◦•————

In almost any medical research encounter—whether a surgical procedure, the sampling of one's DNA for large-scale biorepository research, or any among the countless other possibilities—people are asked to document their willing and informed consent for the procedure about to take place. Despite the problems with informed consent, the existence of these forms is the result of a long, hard-fought struggle against medical paternalism and the regime of usability that justified experimentation on the indigent, the developmentally disabled, and others. Recalling that struggle is the task of bioethical memory, the mobilization of rhetoric's mnestic capacities in order to bear witness to the past. Bioethical memory articulates individuals into the role of witness through *philia* and other emotions, as well as the panoply of material and symbolic supports common to all public memory. Yet, while we are called to witness this history and commit to supporting the systems that prevent the harms of the past, individuals and institutions are often invested in *minimal remembrance,* the crafting of memories sufficient to address a historical and ongoing outcry over the past, yet containing as little detail as possible that could harm an individual's or institution's reputation. The entanglement and contest of bioethical memory and minimal remembrance can be seen in the memory work performed at various sites in response to events in medical research history, specifically the Tuskegee Study of Untreated Syphilis, the Willowbrook Hepatitis Study, and the Cincinnati Whole Body Radiation Study. In this conclusion, I consider some of the implications of the memories and memorials studied here and what they tell us about bioethical memory, minimal remembrance, forgetting, place, and bioethics as a discipline.

Witnesses, Narrative, and Feeling

Public memory offers us narratives that shape our identities in part through the mobilization of public feeling. Those narratives of the past also give form to our ethical impulses. As Arthur Frank reminds us, "Goodness and badness need stories to make them thinkable."[1] Individuals are called to witness the stories from medical research's past. In doing so, they are called to consider the lessons of this past, to name the goodness and the badness made thinkable in those stories. These narratives and the witness role they offer gain power in part because of their mobilization of public feelings. Foremost is the public feeling of philia, the sense of affiliation and belonging. In coming into philia, individuals also develop a sense of *homonoia* or concord: the narrative's contents become the basis for shared judgments and know-how. While philia is an important public feeling, it does not operate alone. As Carole Blair and colleagues argue, scholars must also consider additional public feelings that facilitate philia.[2] In bioethical memory, those ancillary feelings include anger, disgust, and the *unheimlich* or uncanny. Each of these feelings can mobilize one to affiliate as a witness, but each can also have problematic entailments or limits on their effectivity that can play an important role in bioethical public memory.

That potential ambivalence in public feeling shapes the impact of bioethical memory. Take, for example, bioethical memory as it is articulated in the origin story of bioethics shared in medical research training. Stories of medical research and its ethical failures tell medical researchers and bioethicists who they collectively were in order to reassure them that *they are now different.* The ethical failures of the past led to the reforms that shape the present. The story assures students that the worst ethical failures are in the past *for those who adhere to the values of bioethics* as reflected in documents like the Belmont Report. This narrative can potentially open the space for the unheimlich. When researchers hear the warning "That's just like Tuskegee," their affiliation to the position of ethical researcher and witness to past failures accounted for in classroom's instantiation of memory might encourage them to engage in self-reflection, leading to more ethical research. Yet, students might reject the warning "That's just like Tuskegee," believing that the changes to medical research represented by the Belmont Report, IRBs, and bioethics training courses mitigate any need for concern. The feeling of the unheimlich then becomes an unnecessary disturbance of the physician's or researcher's detachment and objectivity.

Similarly, a range of affective responses can occur when individuals encounter the memory narratives offered at the memorials and museums studied here. As differing reactions of anger, disgust, and the unheimlich develop, different degrees and types of philia will arise in visitors as they encounter the call to become witnesses. For example, vernacular memory of Willowbrook evokes disgust and horror at the conditions of the school. These public feelings saturate memory artifacts like the film *Unforgotten* and help affiliate audiences as witnesses who must "never forget" and thus guard against disrespect and disregard for those with developmental disabilities. In the case of Tuskegee, both museums frame the Study as the result of racism. The main difference between the two is that the Tuskegee History Center frames the risks of a recurrence of the Study as unlikely: the lawsuit against the federal government ended those forms of medical racism and ushered us into an era of civil rights. While we must work to maintain that era and its gains, the center's narrative implies that much of the work of bringing the civil rights movement to fruition was accomplished by skilled lawyers in the past. The Legacy Museum emphasizes that a "legacy" of racism persists and requires the ongoing work of many groups, of which Tuskegee University is and was at the forefront. This has differing implications for black and white visitors, as their experiences of race and racism lead to different degrees of anger and (especially white visitors) the potential experience of the uncanny as they find themselves implicated in the racism that led to the Study. Missing from both visions are the complications of class that helped facilitate the Study; the details of how officials from the Tuskegee Institute and other African American institutions enabled the study are absent from the Legacy Museum, and while they can be found at the History Center, the implications of those details are not fully explored.

Another implication of philia and homonoia is that it can militate against bioethical memory narratives. Medical researchers were—and to a degree, still are—constituted by an identity grounded in the tenets of the Hippocratic Oath: Physicians, and medical researchers, believe their purpose is to help the sick, and they believe that in that work they must first do no harm. That identity and the philia clinicians and researchers have for it are so great that medical professionals have resisted the narratives commonly part of bioethical memory. Some physicians claim that the Tuskegee study was not unethical.[3] Historically, physicians fought against outside oversight, especially by the government, believing that it violated the physician-patient and physician–research subject relationships—relationships that were the bedrock of medical ethics. Similarly, we can see this resistance in the work to forget the Cincinnati WBS. The researchers at Cincinnati felt they were doing good science. Senator Kennedy's attack on the study threatened their identity as physicians, grounded as it was in the Hippocratic dictum to "do no harm." Saenger, his research team, and their colleagues at the university's medical school rejected narratives the public crafted about their study because the narratives depicted them as manifestly harming their patient-subjects. Their efforts to reject these narratives in the 1970s and again in the 1990s were successful, whereas the efforts of physicians and researchers involved in Tuskegee were not.[4]

One final observation about public feeling is that when the unheimlich is evoked, it is often done implicitly and subtly. Some stories, like bioethics's origin story or the memory instantiated in the Legacy Museum, might foster a degree of the unheimlich, but the museum's *ennoia* makes it easy for visitors to miss cues that would lead them to experience the unheimlich. The one instance of bioethical memory studied that employs the unheimlich is Ross Cohen's short film *Willowbrook*. Most vernacular memory of Willowbrook emphasizes disgust and horror at the school's conditions. Viewers of memory artifacts like the film *Unforgotten* are called to witness these horrors and commit to the reparative justice project of acknowledging the humanity of the developmentally disabled, which the film situates as the critical step to preventing similar living conditions for the developmentally disabled to arise. Cohen's film, in contrast, allows viewers to experience protagonist Bill Huntsman's experience of the unheimlich through its fantasia of Brian Sussman. The film's audience sees Huntsman come to believe that injecting patients with hepatitis is wrong, although that conclusion does not stop the injections. Yet, to allow viewers to experience Bill's sense of the uncanny, it has to sanitize the conditions at Willowbrook and the conditions of the experiment. To display the uncanny, the film eschews the disgust and horror common to other vernacular memories of Willowbrook. The rarity of the unheimlich in bioethical memory is noteworthy, given the role it supposedly plays in self-reflection and ethical transformation. One possibility is that the unheimlich is a tenuous feeling: Michael Hyde often describes it as stealing up on individuals at odd moments and disturbing their sense of know-how, the concord vitally important to philia. Other strong emotions, like disgust and anger, that orient individuals to the world and to the contents of memory rather than creating the sense of disorientation associated with the unheimlich might fit public memory and bioethical memory better. In other words, the unheimlich might drive individual ethical contemplation, but it does not motivate the public or institutions to act ethically. For that task, other public feelings are required.

Minimal Remembrance, Forgetting,
and the Role of Institutions

The call to witness the times when medicine went wrong is powerful, and it is saturated with public feelings that help that call circulate and persuade. Yet, these memories also represent a threat to various groups and institutions. The responses of those groups can be understood as minimal remembrance and, at its apotheosis, as acts of meaningful forgetting or mnemonicide. While it has similarities to Barbie Zelizer's concept of "remembering to forget," minimal remembrance focuses attention on the role and motivations of institutions in deliberately uncutting memory. Some of the institutions responsible for questionable or horrific events in medical history are also responsible for remembering them, which places their obligation to facilitate memory and witnessing against their need to maintain the institution's reputation and good name. Institutions and groups might be tempted to place their own narratives and organizational memories in the place of bioethical and public memory, but the history of the events that gave birth to bioethics transformed the practice of medicine and medical research, as well as transforming the groups and institutions whose reputations are at stake in bioethical memory. This context—the obligation to remember troubling history and the need to secure one's reputation—is the basic enticement for minimal remembrance.

The case of Willowbrook and official public memory of the school is emblematic of these tendencies. Conditions at Willowbrook were horrific, and official public memory tries to downplay those conditions because blame for them could potentially redound back to New York State for allowing them to persist. Official memories engage in minimal remembrance by using monumental rather than memorial forms to remember the school, thus placing the events firmly in the past, divorced from the present. Official public memory tries to foreclose the reexperiencing of the horror Willowbrook's conditions evoked: They foreclose the middle voice of public memory and place the events at Willowbrook firmly in the past, disconnected from contemporary events. These memories also portray the state as the heroic actor working valiantly to close the school and other large institutions for the developmentally disabled. They ignore that the state was the very entity that created and maintained those institutions, and that the state resisted closing Willowbrook during a ten-year-long legal battle. The monumental mode of memory deployed here sequesters Willowbrook's conditions in the past, treating them as a horror vanquished by the state. This mode avoids the middle voice necessary for animating the past as a concern for the present. While Willowbrook is remembered, most of its past is washed away so that only the singular fact of Willowbrook's closure remains in view.

Sometimes, official memory work moves beyond minimal remembrance and attempts forgetting the events in medical research's past. In the case of Cincinnati, the memories that began developing and circulating were a threat to the identity of the university and its biomedical researchers. As a result, the university actively suppressed the circulation of the memory in the 1970s with the aid of Senator Robert Taft Jr. While a lawsuit settlement forced the university to memorialize the subjects of the study, the memorial fosters forgetting. It is sited in a quasi-public space, the conditions of which indicate to passersby that nothing of note should be there. The memorial is hard to access, and it was only maintained when public outcry called attention to its condition.

That institutional and state actors might suppress embarrassing and shameful events from their past is unsurprising. The actions of New York State and the University of Cincinnati should not surprise, even as they disappoint. This makes the complicated performance of memory at the Tuskegee University Legacy Museum all the more interesting. Here, an institution faces a robust memory culture where the naming of the event—the *Tuskegee* Syphilis Study—is viewed by some as a slight to the institution and the city where it resides. It also hints at broader critiques of the anti-racist action of the institution and its founder Booker T. Washington. Those hints are made explicit, although perhaps not very prominent, at the opposing museum dedicated to the Study. In response to this memory culture and its instantiation at the Tuskegee History Center, the Legacy Museum engages in ennoia: The details and the history of the Study are entirely absent from the site, but the structuring of that absence within the exhibits and space of the Legacy Museum makes the Study, its roots in racism, and the legacy of that racism manifestly present. Visitors to the Legacy Museum traverse a performance of memory emphasizing the lingering legacy of racism, as well as the legacy of fighting racism. While the insinuations that classism and other divides between the Tuskegee Institute/University and the broader Macon County black community are absent, they are not suppressed. Visitors to the Legacy Museum are told about the History Center and its remembrance of the Study, allowing for the performance of memorial agon. While such ennoiatic strategies might not be ideal, they leave open the space for new and innovative performances of memory.

This range of memory practices emphasizes the importance of how rhetoricians and public memory scholars conceptualize practices that minimize or eliminate memory and undercut practices of remembrance. In response to the commonplace framing of public memory as a dialectic of remembering and forgetting, some scholars have questioned the utility of the dialectic, viewing the range of things "forgotten" as so large as to render the remembering-forgetting dialectic meaningless. This charge gains traction when forgetting is framed as *amnesia*. Such a framing is misleading. Instead we should consider public memory as those narratives that "stick" (to borrow Sara Ahmed's language) to publics. That stickiness is the result of investments of public feeling, the circulation of narratives, and the material and symbolic supports for public memory: These saturate specific contents and make them stick in the public's memory. Forgetting, then, would involve making memories "unstick"—removing the material and symbolic supports so that the memory is no longer saturated with public feeling and fails to circulate. Forgetting, then, involves undermining the *publicness* of public memory. Minimal remembrance operates in spaces where events are too sticky—when they are so saturated with public feeling, have circulated widely, and transformed social practices and collective identities. Minimal remembrance keeps what cannot be eliminated (e.g., Willowbrook was a horrible place), while deflecting from aspects of memory that harm an institution's reputation. Sometimes, memory work, especially official memory work, can transform the relationship of institutions and groups to those events.

The examples of remembering, minimal remembrance, and forgetting here also reaffirm the ability of institutions to shape what gets reified in memorials. Institutions' power to shape memory narratives going forward depends on their past ability to control and shape the stories that first brought an event to light. Public memory is drafted over successive rhetorical acts, building on early "drafts" found in journalistic coverage of events as well as the oral histories and other modes of collective memory falling just short of "public memory."[5] When public discourse and shared and collective memories are transformed into public memories, they create multiple, overlapping, and competing threads of public memories that collectively fashion a culture of remembrance around an event. Memorials must reflect that memory culture or be viewed as inauthentic or illegitimate. Forgetting and different modes of remembrance develop as a result of the interaction of existing identities and affective investments with the contents of a memory.

The Power of Place and History

Place and history play important roles in public memory generally and bioethical memory specifically. The designation of a site as a *memory place* indicates the power and resources dedicated to remembering, and it is an indirect indication that groups found some aspect of those events worth remembering. Some of this power is institutional—having the resources to construct a memorial or museum and having the rights to a property that can be converted into a memory place. Yet, that power sometimes comes from social movements, lay groups, and the public: The efforts of non-state actors can give vernacular memories physical form. The Tuskegee History Center and the Building 19 memorial at Willowbrook reflect the efforts of groups—Fred Gray and his supporters in Tuskegee, the people working at the College of Staten Island, respectively—to marshal resources to create their own memory sites or to persuade institutions to create a memory site. The Willowbrook Mile is an attempt to marshal similar support to realize a broader memorial vision.

Memory places have a status as a site of significance because of the costs and effort that go into creating them. Given the general rarity of memory places—and even more so the rarity of memory places devoted to science and medicine—the focus on events where medicine went wrong and led to grave ethical violations is noteworthy. This reflects the importance placed on witnessing and memorializing human rights abuses and other acts of injustice since the late twentieth century. Such witnessing to medicine's failings is an imperative for many. The impact of medical research and its accomplishments in the twentieth century, especially during and after World War II, is staggering. As a result of those accomplishments (and the savvy rhetorical mobilization of that history by physicians and scientists), medicine and medical research is a powerful institution that enters people's lives often when they are most vulnerable. Medicine and medical research's failures, the times where they go wrong, are then all the more terrifying. Given the immense power we give to medicine, its failures demand a restorative justice, of which the witnessing of bioethical memory plays a key part.

Yet public memorials and museums are not the only places where medical research's ethical failures—where it has gone wrong—are displayed. Medical research's ethical failures also appear in the place of the bioethical memory—the classroom. Various regulations from the NIH and the PHS require researchers, especially students and trainees in medical research, to learn about bioethics and the responsible conduct of research. Bioethical memory appears at the beginning of the standard bioethics curriculum as the origin story for bioethics and research regulation. These spaces are multiple and can be both virtual and physical, thus complicating the rhetorical account of the importance of place. While the place as signifier is important because of its rarity and the indication that the place qua place requires significant investment, the bioethical place does not have the same significance.

The lack of investment on a par with public memory places allows more history and other forms of collective memory to be incorporated into the narratives presented in the bioethical place. Teachers of bioethics and responsible conduct of research can add in examples either of local interest or related to the specific types of research conducted at the institution (e.g., pediatric examples for a pediatric hospital, pharmaceutical examples for an RCR course taught to pharmacy students, etc.). New examples—whether the story of Henrietta Lacks, the discovery of the PHS syphilis experiments in Guatemala, or the recently rediscovered World War II mustard gas tests—could be swapped into this opening narrative. Given the history of medical research, there are many examples that could be crowded into this origin story. Yet that very same history makes it unlikely that the major cases of bioethics—the Tuskegee Syphilis Study, the Willowbrook Hepatitis Study, and the less publicly known Jewish Chronic Disease Hospital cancer study—will be crowded out. Unlike other forms of public memory, bioethical memory (especially the bioethics origin story) and history are tightly intertwined; in fact, the origin story is a truncated history. The rhetorical form of the origin story and the history of medical research reinforce each other. The Jewish Chronic Disease Hospital study, while not remembered or marked in public spaces, remains a key part of the bioethics origin story because it represents the event that led the NIH to start regulating medical research and requiring informed consent. It represents the start of the story. Willowbrook exemplifies concerns about research with children and others unable to give informed consent, key concerns for bioethics in the past and present. Finally, the close of the origin story is predetermined and also reflects the historical flow of events: The public revelation of the PHS Study of Untreated Syphilis in Tuskegee helped guarantee the passage of the National Research Act that led to the Belmont Report. These events are given the sense of inevitability in the origin story: For the bioethics classroom and this origin story, these types of atrocities *end* with the Tuskegee Syphilis Study as the event that led to the Belmont Report and subsequent federal regulation of research.

The ending of the bioethical origin story reinforces the tendency of public and bioethical recollection to frame all historical research failings as variations of the Tuskegee Syphilis Study. The study at Tuskegee—or more specifically, the narrative embodied in the naming convention "The Tuskegee Syphilis Study"—represents what Kendall Phillips describes as "the kind of dominant, reified and calcified forms of remembrance that serve to establish broader frameworks within which the fantasies of public memory are contained and proscribed."[6] In some cases, treating a study as a variation on the theme of Tuskegee represents a literal truth: This is the case with the Guatemala syphilis study, where the same researchers worked on both studies, seeking answers to the same research questions. The World War II mustard gas studies are also described as "like Tuskegee," but multiple racial groups—African American, European American, and Asian American—were exposed, unlike Tuskegee where only African American men were observed and had treatment withheld. While some version of scientific and medical racism exists in both studies—both were grounded in the belief that different racial categories would have different disease courses with syphilis and different reactions to mustard gas—and while such racism is troubling and endures in various forms today, the mustard gas study is substantially different from Tuskegee. The syphilis study focused solely on African Americans, took advantage of segregation, and fostered dependence on the Study and limiting the men's access to a cure. None of these qualities holds true for the World War II mustard gas studies.

Complaining about the reframing of these disparate studies as "just like Tuskegee" might seem like a pedant's quibble, but it is a vital recognition of the historical *range of harms* that medical research has inflicted—and still can inflict. The failures of medical research studied here were not purely racist or purely medical. They cut across multiple facets of American life in the mid-twentieth century, some of which endure to this day. Racism and ableism are two dimensions, but underlying them was a larger drive to render *all bodies* usable by the state. If one was not (re)producing, one had to become useful in some other fashion. This helped facilitate studies of cancer with terminal cancer patients, studies of hepatitis among the institutionalized, and studies of syphilis among the segregated and racially oppressed. We live with the history of ableism and racism still today.

Informing Bioethics

So far, I have placed more emphasis on the implications of this project for rhetoric and public memory, including how bioethics complicates some of these issues in rhetorical studies of public memory. Yet the study of bioethical memory also has implications for bioethics and medical research.

First, the research practices that led to medicine going wrong were driven by the combination of medical paternalism and the drive to usability. While usability as it was practiced in the mid-twentieth century no longer exists, the demand to render bodies useful and productive persists. Medical research still renders bodies useful for medical research. This is not nefarious and instead reflects the fact that medicine only develops through testing on bodies. Now, bodies are not coerced or deceived into medical research. The bodies used are those of informed volunteers. Yet, researchers worry about the loss of control: Volunteers always have the right to withdraw from a study, and many who never officially withdraw disappear and are, as researchers say, "lost to follow-up." The demand for the full measure of usability, even from potentially unreliable volunteers, recently led Sarah Edwards to argue that research participants must sign a contract that would lock participants into the full term of a research study and prevent issues like loss to follow-up.[7] The neoliberal language of self-directed economic agents with the full capacity to make individual fully informed choices underlies such proposals, ignoring the degree to which the research enterprise and the burdens it could place on participants remain beyond the knowledge of everyday people. Similarly, a quid pro quo logic underlies commercially available ancestry testing, from companies like 23andMe: You can receive information about yourself for a small fee, but in order to recoup the costs not covered by that fee, your body will be made useful and patentable by the company. The logic of usability persists in these areas, and this persistent logic could contribute to future ethical failures of medical research.

Yet usability alone could not have led to mid-twentieth-century medical practice. Usability operated alongside medical paternalism.

Such paternalism had an ethic of beneficence and non-maleficence (e.g., do good and avoid doing evil), but it sidestepped issues of autonomy and justice. While the systemic support for such paternalism has been undercut, those attitudes still persist and manifest in different ways.[8] Recent scholarship argues that this paternalism has begun manifesting in medical practice concerning genomics. There, clinicians and researchers have begun to move away from a language of "personalized genomic medicine" to "predictive medicine." As Eric Juengst, Michelle McGowan, Jennifer Fishman, and Richard Settersten argue, the language of "personalized genomic medicine" emphasized patient empowerment, but the shift in naming strategies "is a turn away from 'patient empowerment' and toward expert-mediated decision-making in the clinical setting, reviving debates over medical paternalism."[9] Such a shift is even more notable and troubling because it departs from the "traditional ethos of clinical genetics" that has emphasized patient choice and empowerment, a tradition that predates the move toward increased patient autonomy in medical practice generally.[10] For paternalism to arise in a medical specialty that has made patient autonomy and shared decision making foundational highlights the tenacity of medicine's paternalism. That paternalism threatens the values bioethical memories say were secured more than forty years ago, and it does so by undercutting the practices that enable increased autonomy for patients and research participants.

Second, while the events remembered in public places and the events remembered in bioethical places are the same, bioethics would benefit from considering how the content and style of those stories differ, and pay more heed to the public version of these events. All three events considered here raise issues of justice that implicate race, ability, and class. Justice has been a key value in bioethics since the initial publication of Tom Beauchamp and James Childress's *Principles of Biomedical Ethics,* a foundational text for the field.[11] Yet, enacting the commitment to justice has been an ongoing challenge. While there have been recent calls for anti-racist action by bioethicists, those calls have focused primarily on access to health care and not biomedical research.[12] While anti-racist action in bioethics would improve the ethics of medical re-search, such a move would be complicated by how bioethics defines justice in research settings. Both clinical and research bioethics have the same core values of autonomy, beneficence, and justice.[13] The differ-ences lie in the application of justice and its relation to beneficence and autonomy. According to the Belmont Report, the application of justice is limited to the selection of research subjects. On the one hand, this was a profound move by the authors of the Belmont Report: As they note, issues of subject selection had not historically been considered im-portant for medical and scientific ethics. In the United States, indigent patients were routinely used in experiments by medical doctors in the first two-thirds of the twentieth century, because they viewed it as the way patients "paid their way."[14]

While important at the time it was made, the framing of justice as primarily an issue of subject selection is quite limited. The question of how to apply justice to subject selection is seriously underdeveloped in the Report. This becomes clear when discussions of justice are compared to how beneficence and autonomy are operationalized. The Belmont Report identifies processes of informed consent as the practical embodi-ment of autonomy and an elaborate utilitarian calculus of risks and benefits as the way of embodying beneficence in research practice. There is no similar practical embodiment for justice. Even today, the subjects of biomedical research are still overwhelmingly the poorer members of society, although not deceived or coerced as they were at Tuskegee or Willowbrook.[15] In some cases, researchers develop appropriate tools for soliciting informed consent and mitigating potential harms, yet never consider the issues of justice that should lead them to *not* start a research project. This becomes clear in examples like the Kennedy Krieger lead-abatement study: Researchers proposed studying whether partial lead abatement in poorer neighborhoods of Baltimore, Maryland, reduced the amount of lead in the blood of children living in those homes, but partial lead abatement was only considered because landlords in the city were unwilling to incur the expenses of total lead abatement that eliminated childhood lead exposure. In short, poor children were being exposed to lead paint, even at reduced levels, because landlords and the larger society did not want to take on the cost of protecting them.[16]

The memories instantiated at museums and memorials to Tuskegee and Willowbrook—as well as the public outcry against the Cincinnati WBS study—all emphasize concerns about justice related to issues of race, ability, and class. They demand that these concerns be taken seriously, but those concerns require expanding the vision of justice in clinical and research bioethics.

Notes

———•+•———

INTRODUCTION

1. David C. Lindberg, *The Beginnings of Western Science: The European Scientific Tradition in Philosophical, Religious, and Institutional Context, 600 B.C. to A.D. 1450* (Chicago: University of Chicago Press, 1992), 113–31; David J. Rothman, *Strangers at the Bedside* (New York: Basic Books, 1991), 18–19.

2. Susan Lederer, *Subjected to Science: Human Experimentation in America before the Second World War* (Baltimore, MD: Johns Hopkins University Press, 1995), 140–42; Rothman, *Strangers at the Bedside,* 18–29.

3. Rebecca Skloot, *The Immortal Life of Henrietta Lacks,* Kindle e-book ed. (New York: Broadway Books, 2010), 30.

4. This history is drawn primarily from Ruth Faden and Tom L. Beauchamp, *A History and Theory of Informed Consent* (New York: Oxford University Press, 1986), 52–66, 76–100.

5. Henry K. Beecher, "Ethics and Clinical Research," *New England Journal of*

Medicine 274, no. 24 (1966): 1354–60.

6. Stephen B. Thomas and Sandra Crouse Quinn, "Light on the Shadow of the Syphilis Study at Tuskegee," *Health Promotion & Practice* 1, no. 3 (2000): 234.

7. Thomas G. Benedek and Jonathon Erlen, "The Scientific Environment of the Tuskegee Study of Syphilis, 1920–1960," *Perspectives in Biology and Medicine* 43, no. 1 (1999); Robert M. White, "Unraveling the Tuskegee Syphilis Study," *Arthritis Care & Research* 47, no. 4 (2002). For a counter to the arguments made in defense of the study, see Susan M. Reverby, *Examining Tuskegee: The Infamous Syphilis Study and Its Legacy,* reprint (Chapel Hill: University of North Carolina Press, 2009), 230–35.

8. Language of blame and vindication comes from Kendall R. Phillips, "Introduction," in *Framing Public Memory,* ed. Kendall R. Phillips (Tuscaloosa: University of Alabama Press, 2004). Jeffrey K. Olick offers a parallel linguistic framing in his observation that public memory is about shame, responsibility, and regret; Jeffrey K. Olick, *The Politics of Regret: On Collective Memory and Historical Responsibility* (New York: Routledge, 2007).

9. Thomas Kuhn, *The Structure of Scientific Revolutions,* 2nd ed. (Chicago: University of Chicago Press, 1970).

10. Martin Heidegger, *Being and Time,* trans. John Macquarrie and Edward Robinson (New York: Harper & Row, 1962), 233.

11. See Faden and Beauchamp, *History and Theory of Informed Consent,* 86–100; Lederer, *Subjected to Science.*

12. The history in this paragraph comes from a number of essays published on or near the 100th anniversary of the Flexner Report's publication. See Warren D. Anderson, "Outside Looking In: Observations on Medical Education since the Flexner Report," *Medical Education* 45 (2011); Donald A. Barr, "Revolution or Evolution? Putting the Flexner Report in Context," *Medical Education* 45 (2011); Kenneth M. Ludmerer, "Abraham Flexner and Medical Education," *Perspectives in Biology and Medicine* 54, no. 1 (2011); Douglas Page and Adrian Baranchuk, "The Flexner Report: 100 Years Later," *International Journal of Medical Education* 1 (2010). For the impact of increased professionalization on complementary medicine, see Frank W. Stahnisch and Marja Verhoef, "The Flexner Report of 1910 and

Its Impact on Complementary and Alternative Medicine and Psychiatry in North America in the 20th Century," *Evidence-Based Complementary and Alternative Medicine* 2012, Article ID 647896 (2012). For the impact on African American medical education, see Lynn E. Miller and Richard M. Weiss, "Revisiting Black Medical School Extinctions in the Flexner Era," *Journal of the History of Medicine and Allied Sciences* 67, no. 2 (2011).

13. James H. Jones, *Bad Blood: The Tuskegee Syphilis Experiment* (New York: Free Press, 1993), 95.

14. Jones, *Bad Blood,* 97.

15. Lederer, *Subjected to Science,* xv. Lederer is partly responding to Jones, who argued that the lack of an enforceable code led to a "formless relativism." See Jones, *Bad Blood,* 97.

16. Lisa Keränen, "The Hippocratic Oath as Epideictic Rhetoric: Reanimating Medicine's Past for Its Future," *Journal of Medical Humanities* 22, no. 1 (2001). While it is often spoken of as a singular thing, Keränen notes that no single version of the Oath exists or is in use. Claims about "what the Oath contains or lacks" reflect trends across the extant versions in use during the modern era.

17. Keränen, "The Hippocratic Oath," 60.

18. Jordan Goodman, Anthony McElligott, and Lara Marks, "Making Human Bodies Useful: Historicizing Medical Experiments in the Twentieth Century," in *Useful Bodies,* ed. Jordan Goodman, Anthony McElligott, and Lara Marks (Baltimore, MD: Johns Hopkins University Press, 2003), 2.

19. Goodman, McElligott, and Marks, "Making Human Bodies Useful," 12n54.

20. Rothman, *Strangers at the Bedside,* 3–4.

21. E.g., "Secret World War II Chemical Experiments Tested Troops by Race," *NPR Morning Edition,* June 22, 2015, available at www.npr.org/2015/06/22/415194765/u-s-troops-tested-by-race-in-secret-world-war-ii-chemical-experiments.

CHAPTER 1. BIOETHICAL MEMORY AND MINIMAL REMEMBRANCE

1. Carole Blair, Greg Dickinson, and Brian L. Ott, "Introduction: Rhetoric/Memory/Place," in *Places of Public Memory: The Rhetoric of Museums and Memorials,* ed. Greg Dickinson, Carole Blair, and Brian L. Ott (Tuscaloosa: University of Alabama Press, 2010), 5–6.

2. Thomas R. Dunn, "Remembering 'a Great Fag': Visualizing Public Memory and the Construction of Queer Space," *Quarterly Journal of Speech* 97, no. 4 (2011): 439.

3. Nathan Stormer, *Sign of Pathology: U.S. Medical Rhetoric on Abortion, 1800s–1960s* (University Park, PA: Penn State University Press, 2015), 49–53.

4. The range of public memory artifacts studied by rhetoricians is captured by this partial, yet representative list: Stephen Browne, "Reading Public Memory in Daniel Webster's *Plymouth Rock Oration,*" *Western Journal of Communication* 57 (1993); Thomas R. Dunn, "Remembering Matthew Shepard: Violence, Identity and Queer Counterpublic Memories," *Rhetoric & Public Affairs* 13, no. 4 (2010); Kristen Hoerl, "Burning Mississippi into Memory: Cinematic Amnesia as a Resource for Civil Rights," *Critical Studies in Media Communication* 26, no. 1 (2009); John A. Lynch, "Memory and Matthew Shepard: Opposing Expressions of Public Memory in Television Movies," *Journal of Communication Inquiry* 31, no. 3 (2007); Charles E. Morris III, "My Old Kentucky Homo: Lincoln and the Politics of Queer Public Memory," in *Framing Public Memory,* ed. Kendall R. Phillips (Tuscaloosa: University of Alabama Press, 2004); Bradford J. Vivian, "Jefferson's Other," *Quarterly Journal of Speech* 88 (2002); Barbie Zelizer, *Remembering to Forget: Holocaust Memory through the Camera's Lens* (Chicago: University of Chicago Press, 1998).

   The focus on memorials and museums can be seen in a range of work including Greg Dickinson, Brian L. Ott, and Eric Aoki, "Memory and Myth at the Buffalo Bill Museum," *Western Journal of Communication* 69, no. 2 (2005); Greg Dickinson, Brian L. Ott, and Eric Aoki, "Spaces of Remembering and Forgetting: The Reverent Eye/I at the Plains Indian Museum," *Communication and Critical/Cultural Studies* 3, no. 1 (2006); Dunn, "Remembering 'a Great Fag'"; Victoria J. Gallagher, "Memory and Reconciliation in the Birmingham Civil Rights Institute," *Rhetoric & Public*

Affairs 2, no. 2 (1999); Marouf Hasian Jr., "Remembering and Forgetting the "Final Solution": A Rhetorical Pilgrimage to the Holocaust Museum," *Critical Studies in Media Communication* 21, no. 1 (2004); Tamar Katriel, "Sites of Memory: Discourses of the Past in Israeli Pioneering Settlement Museums," *Quarterly Journal of Speech* 80, no. 1 (1994); Charles E. Morris III, ed. *Remembering the AIDS Quilt* (East Lansing: Michigan State University Press, 2011); Brian L. Ott, Eric Aoki, and Greg Dickinson, "Ways of (Not) Seeing Guns: Presence and Absence at the Cody Firearms Museum," *Communication & Critical/Cultural Studies* 8, no. 3 (2011).

5. Blair, Dickinson, and Ott, "Introduction," 6; Barbie Zelizer, "Reading the Past against the Grain: The Shape of Memory Studies," *Critical Studies in Mass Communication* 12 (1995): 224. Historian Susan Reverby highlights the partiality of various memory artifacts devoted to the Tuskegee Study; see "Introduction: More Than a Metaphor: An Overview of the Scholarship of the Study," in *Tuskegee's Truths: Rethinking the Tuskegee Syphilis Study,* ed. Susan M. Reverby (Chapel Hill: University of North Carolina Press, 2000), 1.

6. Zelizer, *Remembering to Forget,* 10. Zelizer's definition presumes witnessing does not necessarily require a person to have actually observed the events witnessed, an assumption made explicit recently in the work of Brad Vivian; see Bradford J. Vivian, *Commonplace Witnessing: Rhetorical Invention, Historical Remembrance, and Public Culture* (New York: Oxford University Press, 2017).

7. Vivian, *Commonplace Witnessing,* 11.

8. Zelizer, *Remembering to Forget,* 10.

9. Arthur W. Frank, "Truth Telling, Companionship and Witness: An Agenda for Narrative Bioethics," *Hastings Center Report* 46, no. 3 (2016): 20. Other narrative bioethicists frame the mission of bioethics more broadly as a focus on how narratives organize and evaluate the world while also vivifying ethical commitments; see Howard Brody and Mark Clark, "Narrative Ethics: A Narrative," *Hastings Center Report* 44, no. 1 (2014); Martha Montello, "Narrative Ethics," *Hastings Center Report* 44, no. 1 (2014).

10. Blair, Dickinson, and Ott, "Introduction," 7.

11. Marouf Hasian, "Authenticity, Public Memories, and the Problematics of Post-Holocaust Remembrances: A Rhetorical Analysis of the Wilkomirski Affair," *Quarterly Journal of Speech* 91, no. 3 (2005): 256.

12. Edward S. Casey, "Public Memory in Place and Time," in *Framing Public Memory,* ed. Kendall R. Phillips (Tuscaloosa: University of Alabama Press, 2004), 29.

13. Tasha Dubriwny and Kristan Poirot, eds., "Gender and Public Memory," special issue, *Southern Communication Journal* 82, no. 4 (2017); G. Mitchell Reyes, ed., *Public Memory, Race, and Ethnicity* (Newcastle upon Tyne, UK: Cambridge Scholars Publishing, 2010).

14. Jeffrey K. Olick, *The Politics of Regret: On Collective Memory and Historical Responsibility* (New York: Routledge, 2007; Kendall R. Phillips, ed., *Framing Public Memory* (Tuscaloosa: University of Alabama Press, 2004). The concern about responsibility and blame is also emphasized by James H. Jones in relation to bioethical recall of Tuskegee; see James H. Jones, "Foreword," in *Tuskegee's Truths: Rethinking the Tuskegee Syphilis Study,* ed. Susan M. Reverby (Chapel Hill: University of North Carolina Press, 2000), xiii.

15. Blair, Dickinson, and Ott, "Introduction," 14.

16. Debra Hawhee, "Rhetoric's Sensorium," *Quarterly Journal of Speech* 101, no. 1 (2015); Jenell Johnson, "'A Man's Mouth Is His Castle': The Midcentury Fluoridation Controversy and the Visceral Public," *Quarterly Journal of Speech* 102, no. 1 (2016). Hawhee and Johnson draw from the work of Ann Cvetkovich in choosing this term; see Ann Cvetkovich, *Depression: A Public Feeling* (Durham, NC: Duke University Press, 2012).

17. Brian Massumi, *Parables for the Virtual: Movement, Affect, Sensation* (Durham, NC: Duke University Press, 2002).

18. Hawhee, "Rhetoric's Sensorium," 12.

19. Johnson, "A Man's Mouth Is His Castle," 3.

20. Sara Ahmed, *The Cultural Politics of Emotion* (New York: Routledge, 2004). See also Blair, Dickinson, and Ott, "Introduction," 15.

21. Blair, Dickinson, and Ott, "Introduction," 16.

22. Blair, Dickinson, and Ott, "Introduction," 16.

23. Eugene Garver, *Aristotle's Rhetoric: An Art of Character* (Chicago: University of

Chicago Press, 1994), 115–16.

24. In this sense of being indispensable, then, philia becomes something like Martin Heidegger's Being-with-Others; see Heidegger, *Being and Time,* trans. John Macquarrie and Edward Robinson (New York: Harper & Row, 1962), 149–57.

25. Eleni Leontsini, "The Motive of Society: Aristotle on Civic Friendship, Justice, and Concord," *Res Publica* 19, no. 1 (2013): 21.

26. Garver, *Aristotle's Rhetoric;* Leontsini, "Motive of Society"; Robert R. Williams, "Aristotle and Hegel on Recognition and Friendship," in *The Plural States of Recognition,* ed. Michel Seymour (New York: Palgrave Macmillan, 2010).

27. Garver, *Aristotle's Rhetoric,* 32.

28. Garver, *Aristotle's Rhetoric,* 118.

29. Ahmed, *Cultural Politics of Emotion,* 88.

30. Ahmed, *Cultural Politics of Emotion,* 90.

31. Ahmed, *Cultural Politics of Emotion,* 98.

32. Ahmed, *Cultural Politics of Emotion,* 99.

33. Ahmed, *Cultural Politics of Emotion,* 176.

34. Ahmed, *Cultural Politics of Emotion,* 175.

35. Michael J. Hyde, *The Call of Conscience: Heidegger and Levinas, Rhetoric and the Euthanasia Debate* (Columbia: University of South Carolina Press, 2001), 52.

36. Hyde, *Call of Conscience,* 52.

37. Greg Dickinson, *Suburban Dreams: Imagining and Building the Good Life* (Tuscaloosa: University of Alabama Press, 2015), 24–25.

38. Dickinson, *Suburban Dreams,* 187.

39. Jodi Halpern, "What Is Clinical Empathy?," *Journal of General Internal Medicine* 18, no. 8 (2003); Charles Kadushin, "Social Distance between Client and Professional," *American Journal of Sociology* 67, no. 5 (1962); Wei-Ting Tseng and Ya-Ping Lin, "'Detached Concern' of Medical Students in a Cadaver Dissection Course: A Phenomenological Study," *Anatomical Sciences Education* 9, no. 3 (2015).

40. Rosa Eberly, "'Everywhere You Go, It's There': Forgetting and Remembering the University of Texas Tower Shooting," in *Framing Public*

Memory, ed. Kendall R. Phillips (Tuscaloosa: University of Alabama Press, 2004), 71.

41. Barbie Zelizer, "The Voice of the Visual in Memory," in *Framing Public Memory,* ed. Kendall R. Phillips (Tuscaloosa: University of Alabama Press, 2004), 162.

42. Charles E. Scott, "The Appearance of Public Memory," in *Framing Public Memory,* ed. Kendall R. Phillips (Tuscaloosa: University of Alabama Press, 2004), 148–49.

43. Casey, "Public Memory," 32.

44. Blair, Dickinson, and Ott, "Introduction," 25.

45. Elizabethada A. Wright, "Rhetorical Spaces in Memorial Places: The Cemetery as a Rhetorical Space/Place," *Rhetoric Society Quarterly* 25, no. 4 (2005): 71.

46. Blair, Dickinson, and Ott, "Introduction," 27–28.

47. Blair, Dickinson, and Ott, "Introduction," 26. See also Casey, "Public Memory"; Dickinson, Ott, and Aoki, "Spaces of Remembering and Forgetting."

48. Casey, "Public Memory," 25, 37; Kendall R. Phillips, "The Failure of Memory: Reflections on Rhetoric and Public Remembrance," *Western Journal of Communication* 74, no. 2 (2010): 220.

49. Blair, Dickinson, and Ott, "Introduction," 27.

50. See Reverby, *Examining Tuskegee,* chapter 10.

51. For the language of official versus vernacular, see John Bodnar, *Remaking America: Public Memory, Commemoration, and Patriotism in the Twentieth Century* (Princeton, NJ: Princeton University Press, 1992); Stephen Browne, "Reading, Rhetoric and Texture of Public Memory," *Quarterly Journal of Speech* 81 (1995); Zelizer, "Reading the Past against the Grain."

52. Dunn, "Remembering Matthew Shepard," 614.

53. Zelizer, *Remembering to Forget,* 203.

54. Zelizer, *Remembering to Forget,* 202.

55. Kerwin Lee Klein, "On the Emergence of Memory in Historical Discourse," *Representations* 69 (2000); Jeffrey K. Olick, "Collective Memory: The Two Cultures," *Sociological Theory* 17, no. 3 (1999).

56. Olick, "Collective Memory," 335.

57. Casey, "Public Memory," 21.

58. Casey, "Public Memory," 23.

59. Casey, "Public Memory," 23.

60. Casey, "Public Memory," 25.

61. Casey, "Public Memory," 25.

62. Blair, Dickinson, and Ott, "Introduction," 6.

63. Reverby, *Examining Tuskegee,* 193.

64. Klein, "On the Emergence of Memory," 128.

65. Kendall Phillips, "Introduction," in *Framing Public Memory,* ed. Kendall R. Phillips (Tuscaloosa: University of Alabama Press, 2004), 2.

66. Barry Schwartz and Howard Schuman, "History, Commemoration, and Belief: Abraham Lincoln in American Memory, 1945–2001," *American Sociological Review* 70 (2005); Olick, *The Politics of Regret,* 150; Blair, Dickinson, and Ott, "Introduction," 9; Kirt H. Wilson, "Debating the Great Emancipator: Abraham Lincoln and Our Public Memory," *Rhetoric & Public Affairs* 13, no. 3 (2010); Charles E. Morris III, "Sunder the Children: Abraham Lincoln's Queer Rhetorical Pedagogy," *Quarterly Journal of Speech* 99, no. 4 (2013).

67. Marita Sturken, *Tangled Memories* (Berkeley: University of California Press, 1997), 3.

68. Reverby, *Examining Tuskegee,* 188.

69. Reverby, *Examining Tuskegee,* 188.

70. David Thelan, "Memory and American History," *Journal of American History* 75 (1989): 1120.

71. Browne, "Reading, Rhetoric and Texture of Public Memory," 242. See also Phillips, "Introduction," 5–6; Sturken, *Tangled Memories,* 7–9; Zelizer, "Reading the Past against the Grain," 220; Bradford J. Vivian, *Public Forgetting: The Rhetoric and Politics of Beginning Again* (State College, PA: Penn State University Press, 2010).

72. Blair, Dickinson, and Ott, "Introduction," 18.

73. Blair, Dickinson, and Ott, "Introduction," 20.

74. Dickinson, *Suburban Dreams,* 127–31.

75. This conceptual framing is borrowed from Phillips, "Introduction."

76. Blair, Dickinson, and Ott, "Introduction," 19.

77. Vivian, *Public Forgetting,* 46.
78. Vivian, *Public Forgetting,* 46–47.
79. John A. Lynch and Mary E. Stuckey, "'This Was His Georgia': Polio, Poverty, and Public Memory at FDR's Little White House," *Howard Journal of Communication* (2017); Kristan Poirot and Shevaun E. Watson, "Memories of Freedom and White Resilience: Place, Tourism, and Urban Slavery," *Rhetoric Society Quarterly* 45, no. 2 (2015).

Chapter 2. Experiment or Treatment?
Histories of Medical Care, Research, and Regulation

1. Ruth Faden and Tom L. Beauchamp, *A History and Theory of Informed Consent* (New York: Oxford University Press, 1986), 151.
2. David C. Lindberg, *The Beginnings of Western Science: The European Scientific Tradition in Philosophical, Religious, and Institutional Context, 600 B.C. to A.D. 1450* (Chicago: University of Chicago Press, 1992), 113–31; David J. Rothman, *Strangers at the Bedside* (New York: Basic Books, 1991), 18–19.
3. Lindberg, *The Beginnings of Western Science,* 113–31; Rothman, *Strangers at the Bedside,* 18–19.
4. Susan Lederer, *Subjected to Science: Human Experimentation in America before the Second World War* (Baltimore, MD: Johns Hopkins University Press, 1995), 4.
5. Donald A. Barr, "Revolution or Evolution? Putting the Flexner Report in Context," *Medical Education* 45 (2011); Kenneth M. Ludmerer, "Abraham Flexner and Medical Education," *Perspectives in Biology and Medicine* 54, no. 1 (2011).
6. Lederer, *Subjected to Science,* 6.
7. This history is drawn from Faden and Beauchamp, *History and Theory of Informed Consent* 151–52; Lederer, *Subjected to Science,* 4–15; Rothman, *Strangers at the Bedside,* 18–23.
8. Lederer, *Subjected to Science,* 9.
9. Faden and Beauchamp, *History and Theory of Informed Consent,* 61.
10. Lederer, *Subjected to Science,* 18. See also Rebecca Dresser, "Personal Knowledge and Study Participation," *Journal of Medical Ethics* 40 (2014);

Rothman, *Strangers at the Bedside,* 21.

11. This story is drawn from Rebecca M. Herzig, *Suffering for Science: Reason and Sacrifice in Modern America* (New Brunswick, NJ: Rutgers University Press, 2005), 1–2; Lederer, *Subjected to Science,* 19–21; Rothman, *Strangers at the Bedside,* 25–27.

12. Herzig, *Suffering for Science;* see also Lederer, *Subjected to Science,* 126–38.

13. Rothman, *Strangers at the Bedside,* 28.

14. Lederer, *Subjected to Science,* 110.

15. Lederer, *Subjected to Science,* 106.

16. Lederer, *Subjected to Science,* 28; see also Rothman, *Strangers at the Bedside,* 29.

17. Lederer, *Subjected to Science,* xiv.

18. Lederer, *Subjected to Science,* 73.

19. Lederer, *Subjected to Science,* 73–75; Faden and Beauchamp, *A History and Theory of Informed Consent,* 84–86. For more information on quackery, see Lydia Kang and Nate Pedersen, *Quackery: A Brief History of the Worst Ways to Cure Everything* (New York: Workman Publishing Co., 2017); James Harvey Young, *The Medical Messiahs: A Social History of Health Quackery in the Twentieth Century,* expanded paperback ed. (Princeton, NJ: Princeton University Press, 1992).

20. Many histories of research ethics and medical regulation implicitly or explicitly frame World War II as the watershed moment in this history, either by beginning in 1946 or making claims for a radical transformation in medicine at this time; see Advisory Committee on Human Radiation Experiments (ACHRE), *Final Report* (Washington, DC: U.S. Government Printing Office, 1995), 81–170; Faden and Beauchamp, *A History and Theory of Informed Consent;* Rothman *Strangers at the Bedside.* I agree with Susan Lederer that any change that occurred from pre-WWII to post-WWII research was a matter of degree and not one of kind.

21. Rothman, *Strangers at the Bedside,* 31.

22. Rexmond C. Cochrane, *The National Academy of Sciences: The First Hundred Years, 1863–1963* (Washington, DC: National Academies Press, 1978), 410. Rothman states that the CMR expended more than $25 million; *Strangers at the Bedside,* 31.

23. Lederer, *Subjected to Science,* 140; Rothman, *Strangers at the Bedside,* 39–40.

24. Cochrane, *The National Academy of Sciences,* 410–11; Lederer, *Subjected to Science,* 140.

25. Rothman, *Strangers at the Bedside,* 32–38.

26. Lederer, *Subjected to Science,* 140.

27. Leah Ceccarelli, *On the Frontier of Science: An American Rhetoric of Exploration and Exploitation* (East Lansing: Michigan State University Press, 2013), 43–49; Rothman, *Strangers at the Bedside,* 52–53.

28. For more on human radiation experiments, see chapter 5.

29. Faden and Beauchamp, *A History and Theory of Informed Consent,* 153. Faden and Beauchamp wrote this before Japan's Unit 731 and its experimentation on Chinese prisoners and Allied POWs became common knowledge. Those experiments were just as, if not more, horrible, but unlike the Nazi doctors, the Japanese researchers received immunity from prosecution in exchange for giving their data to the United States government; see Sheldon H. Harris, *Factories of Death: Japanese Biological Warfare, 1932–45, and the American Cover-up* (New York: Routledge, 1994).

30. Faden and Beauchamp, *A History and Theory of Informed Consent,* 153.

31. For the ten principles of the Nuremberg Code, see ACHRE, *Final Report,* 103. For more on the trials and the code, see ibid., 131–35; Faden and Beauchamp, *A History and Theory of Informed Consent,* 153–56.

32. ACHRE, *Final Report,* 134–37; Lederer, *Subjected to Science,* 140.

33. ACHRE, *Final Report,* 135–36.

34. ACHRE, *Final Report,* 92.

35. ACHRE, *Final Report,* 105–7.

36. ACHRE, *Final Report,* 114–15; Charles R. McCarthy, "The Origins and Policies That Govern Institutional Review Boards," in *The Oxford Textbook of Clinical Research Ethics,* ed. Ezekiel Emmanuel et al. (New York: Oxford University Press, 2011); Rothman, *Strangers at the Bedside,* 54–58.

37. ACHRE, *Final Report,* 114; see also John C. Fletcher, "Clinical Bioethics at the NIH: History and a New Vision," *Kennedy Institute of Ethics Journal* 5, no. 4 (1995); McCarthy, "Origins and Policies," 543.

38. ACHRE, *Final Report,* 113.

39. McCarthy, "Origins and Policies," 543.

40. Rothman, *Strangers at the Bedside,* 55.

41. ACHRE, *Final Report,* 110.

42. Rothman, *Strangers at the Bedside,* 63.

43. Allen M. Brandt and Lara Freidenfelds, "Research Ethics after World War II: The Insular Culture of Biomedicine," *Kennedy Institute of Ethics Journal* 6, no. 3 (1996): 241.

44. ACHRE, *Final Report,* 149; see also Rothman, *Strangers at the Bedside,* 1–2.

45. Rothman, *Strangers at the Bedside,* 57.

46. ACHRE, *Final Report,* 110, 114.

47. Faden and Beauchamp, *History and Theory of Informed Consent,* 87, 161; Rothman, *Strangers at the Bedside,* 99–100.

48. ACHRE, *Final Report,* 173; Faden and Beauchamp, *History and Theory of Informed Consent,* 203; James E. Ridings, "The Thalidomide Disaster: Lessons from the Past," in *Teratogenicity Testing,* vol. 947, *Methods in Molecular Biology (Methods and Protocols),* ed. Paul C. Barrow (Totowa, NJ: Humana Press, 2013); Rothman, *Strangers at the Bedside,* 63–64.

49. ACHRE, *Final Report,* 173.

50. Faden and Beauchamp, *History and Theory of Informed Consent,* 161.

51. Faden and Beauchamp, *History and Theory of Informed Consent,* 161.

52. John D. Arras, "The Jewish Chronic Disease Hospital Case," in *The Oxford Textbook of Clinical Research Ethics,* ed. Ezekiel Emmanuel et al. (New York: Oxford University Press, 2011), 74.

53. Arras, "The Jewish Chronic Disease Hospital Case," 74–75; Faden and Beauchamp, *History and Theory of Informed Consent,* 161.

54. ACHRE, *Final Report,* 174.

55. Arras, "The Jewish Chronic Disease Hospital Case," 78.

56. Rothman, *Strangers at the Bedside,* 89.

57. ACHRE, *Final Report,* 176.

58. Rothman, *Strangers at the Bedside,* 90.

59. Faden and Beauchamp, *History and Theory of Informed Consent,* 161; Lara Freidenfelds, "Recruiting Allies for Reform: Henry Knowles Beecher's 'Ethics and Clinical Research,'" *International Anesthesiology Clinics* 45, no. 4 (2007); David S. Jones, Christine C. Grady, and Susan E. Lederer, "'Ethics and Clinical Research'—the 50th Anniversary of Beecher's

Bombshell," *New England Journal of Medicine* 374 (2016); Rothman, *Strangers at the Bedside,* 70–76.

60. Rothman, *Strangers at the Bedside,* 75.
61. Jones, Grady, and Lederer, "Ethics and Clinical Research," 2395; see also Rothman, *Strangers at the Bedside,* 75–78.
62. Freidenfelds, "Recruiting Allies for Reform," 85.
63. Rothman, *Strangers at the Bedside,* 82. See also Faden and Beauchamp, *History and Theory of Informed Consent,* 159; Freidenfelds, "Recruiting Allies for Reform," 81.
64. Krugman's research was example 16 in Beecher's article; see Rothman, *Strangers at the Bedside,* 77. More detail on the study can be found in chapter 4.
65. Faden and Beauchamp, *History and Theory of Informed Consent,* 163.
66. For details on how the study escaped attention of early bioethicists, see Susan M. Reverby, *Examining Tuskegee: The Infamous Syphilis Study and Its Legacy,* reprint (Chapel Hill: University of North Carolina Press, 2009), 190–91.
67. See Reverby, *Examining Tuskegee,* 91.
68. Faden and Beauchamp, *History and Theory of Informed Consent,* 166.
69. Faden and Beauchamp, *History and Theory of Informed Consent,* 166–67; Reverby, *Examining Tuskegee,* 91–100. Reverby also discusses limitations on the panel's deliberations. The committee lacked access to early records of the study that would have shown deliberate deception by the PHS doctors from the outset. DHEW also prevented the committee from having a broader discussion of race and racism in medical research and clinical care.
70. Faden and Beauchamp, *History and Theory of Informed Consent,* 167; Rothman, *Strangers at the Bedside,* 183.
71. Rothman, *Strangers at the Bedside,* 168.
72. Rothman, *Strangers at the Bedside,* 169.
73. Rothman, *Strangers at the Bedside,* 183.
74. Reverby, *Examining Tuskegee,* 100–102.
75. Rothman, *Strangers at the Bedside,* 184.
76. Rothman, *Strangers at the Bedside,* 247.

77. ACHRE, *Final Report,* 181.
78. Reverby, *Examining Tuskegee,* 190.
79. Jeffrey M. Cohen, "History and Ethics of Human Subjects Research," CITI Program, https://www.citiprogram.org.

CHAPTER 3. LAWSUITS AND LEGACIES:

COMPETING MEMORIALIZATIONS OF THE TUSKEGEE SYPHILIS STUDY

1. Jean Heller, "Syphilis Victims in U.S. Study Went Untreated for 40 Years," in *Tuskegee's Truths: Rethinking the Tuskegee Syphilis Study,* ed. Susan M. Reverby (Chapel Hill: University of North Carolina Press, 2000). Heller's article first appeared in the *Washington Post.* The number of men in the Study and whether they had syphilis or were a nonsyphilitic control have varied across reports. Most report a number of around 600, with 399 men having latent stage syphilis and 201 controls. The historical details outlined in the remainder of the introduction are drawn from the following sources: Fred D. Gray, *The Tuskegee Syphilis Study: The Real Story and Beyond* (Montgomery, AL: NewSouth Books, 1998); James H. Jones, *Bad Blood: The Tuskegee Syphilis Experiment* (New York: Free Press, 1993); Susan M. Reverby, *Examining Tuskegee: The Infamous Syphilis Study and Its Legacy,* repr. (Chapel Hill: University of North Carolina Press, 2009); Susan M. Reverby, "More Than Fact and Fiction: Cultural Memory and the Tuskegee Syphilis Study," *Hastings Center Report* 31, no. 5 (2001).

2. During the 1930s, syphilis was treated with injections of arsenic and mercury derivatives over the course of months or years before the PHS developed a rapid treatment protocol used in conjunction with the draft for WWII. After the discovery of penicillin, questions about whether those with *latent* syphilis, who were supposedly unable to transmit the disease, should be treated with penicillin persisted through the early 1950s because of potential side effects of the treatment. See Jones, *Bad Blood,* 45–46; Reverby, *Examining Tuskegee,* 3–4, 137, 147; Reverby, "More Than Fact and Fiction," 25–26.

3. James Jones attributes this line to James B. Lucas, who in 1970 was the assistant director of the PHS's Venereal Disease Branch. He also uses the quotation as the title for the tenth chapter of his book; see Jones, *Bad*

Blood, 202.

4. Reverby, "More Than Fact and Fiction," 22.
5. The public naming practice was facilitated by the eventual inclusion of "Tuskegee" in the title of PHS reports about the Study, starting in 1954. See Reverby, *Examining Tuskegee,* 85; Susan M. Reverby, "Invoking 'Tuskegee': Problems in Health Disparities, Genetic Assumptions, and History," *Journal of Health Care for the Poor and Underserved* 21 (2010): 26; Sidney Olansky, Lloyd Simpson, and Stanley H. Schuman, "Environmental Factors in the Tuskegee Study of Untreated Syphilis," *Public Health Reports* 69, no. 7 (1954).
6. Stephen B. Thomas and Sandra Crouse Quinn, "Light on the Shadow of the Syphilis Study at Tuskegee," *Health Promotion & Practice* 1, no. 3 (2000): 236.
7. In addition to the other citations in this paragraph, see Lynn M. Harter, Ronald J. Stephens, and Phyllis M. Japp, "President Clinton's Apology for the Tuskegee Syphilis Experiment: A Narrative of Remembrance, Redefinition and Reconciliation," *Howard Journal of Communications* 11 (2000); Reverby, *Examining Tuskegee;* Susan M. Reverby, "Listening to Narratives from the Tuskegee Syphilis Study," *The Lancet* 377 (2011).
8. Reverby's book was published before the Legacy Museum was built, but she also had a role in helping plan for the Bioethics Center and the Legacy Museum that is a part of it.
9. Reverby, *Examining Tuskegee,* 188.
10. Reverby, *Examining Tuskegee,* 193.
11. Thomas and Quinn, "Light on the Shadow," 236. Reverby makes a similar argument when she describes Tuskegee "as a one-word epithet"; see Reverby, "Listening to Narratives," 1646.
12. Reverby, *Examining Tuskegee,* 188.
13. Reverby, *Examining Tuskegee,* 193; emphasis mine. This deflection of race and racism most clearly occurs in government-sponsored reports on research, like the Belmont Report, and teaching materials in bioethics. Some bioethicists in their research writings have emphasized the role of racism, but those considerations are never translated from bioethical research to bioethical teaching; see Allen M. Brandt, "Racism and

Research: The Case of the Tuskegee Syphilis Experiment," in *Tuskegee's Truths: Rethinking the Tuskegee Syphilis Study,* ed. Susan M. Reverby (Chapel Hill: University of North Carolina Press, 2000).

14. Reverby, *Examining Tuskegee,* 192.
15. Reverby, *Examining Tuskegee,* 193. This has also been my experience when teaching students in biomedical research about Tuskegee. From 2008 to 2014, I taught a "responsible conduct of research" course at the University of Cincinnati medical school. Despite my best efforts, many students did not think Tuskegee applied to them and their work. It was historically too distant and the actions of the researchers so far outside the pale of what they understood as "research."
16. Reverby, "More Than Fact and Fiction," 25.
17. Reverby, "Invoking 'Tuskegee,'" 26. Thompson and Quinn describe it as part of the "folklore of racism"; "Light on the Shadow," 236.
18. Jones, *Bad Blood,* 216. Fred Gray's account of the Study and the lawsuit only identifies two individual PHS officers: John Heller and Sydney Olansky; see Gray, *The Tuskegee Syphilis Study,* 85.
19. Jones, *Bad Blood,* 217; Gray, *The Tuskegee Syphilis Study,* 97–99.
20. Gray, *The Tuskegee Syphilis Study,* 84; Jones, *Bad Blood,* 217.
21. Gray, *The Tuskegee Syphilis Study,* 87–88.
22. Jones, *Bad Blood,* 216; see also Reverby, *Examining Tuskegee,* 106. This choice might seem odd to some, given that the initial reports in 1972 highlighted the role of the Tuskegee Institute and prominently featured Eunice Rivers Laurie, the African American public health nurse tasked by the PHS with maintaining the relationship between the men and the Study. It might also seem like a conflict of interest, since Gray at the time was Tuskegee Institute's general counsel; see Jones, *Bad Blood,* 216. Gray argues that both Tuskegee Institute and Eunice Rivers Laurie were powerless to influence the Study and were as much victims as the men in it, and Susan Reverby argues, "One could hardly imagine Fred Gray doing anything else. Gray did not need anyone to tell him how race, class, and power worked in Alabama"; Reverby, *Examining Tuskegee,* 106.
23. Reverby, *Examining Tuskegee,* 108.
24. Reverby, *Examining Tuskegee,* 133.

25. Jones, *Bad Blood,* chapter 14; Reverby, *Examining Tuskegee,* 199–200; Thompson and Quinn, "Light on the Shadow"; Thompson and Quinn, "The Tuskegee Syphilis Study, 1932–1972: Implications for HIV Education and Aids Risk Education Programs in the Black Community." In *Tuskegee's Truths: Rethinking the Tuskegee Syphilis Study,* ed. Susan M. Reverby (Chapel Hill: University of North Carolina Press, 2000), 404–17.

26. Reverby, *Examining Tuskegee,* 200.

27. Booker T. Washington, "Cotton States Exposition Address," in *American Rhetorical Discourse,* ed. Ronald F. Reid (Prospect Heights, IL: Waveland Press, 1995), 566. Recently, Paul Stob argued that Washington's speech, and this line particularly, is not the capitulation to segregation many believe it is; see Paul Stob, "Black Hands Push Back: Reconsidering the Rhetoric of Booker T. Washington," *Quarterly Journal of Speech* 104, no. 2 (2018).

28. Reverby, *Examining Tuskegee,* 16. This attempt to dissociate himself and the Institute from negative stereotypes of African Americans by emphasizing class distinctions failed. As Reverby noted, Washington himself was unable to escape accusations of sexual licentiousness: When he collapsed in 1915 from arteriosclerosis, high blood pressure, and kidney disease, physicians implied that it was actually due to a history of syphilis; see Reverby, *Examining Tuskegee,* 16–17.

29. W. E. B. Du Bois, *The Souls of Black Folk* (New York: Dover, 1994). Manning Marable argues that Washington's vision remained the primary political philosophy of the Tuskegee Institute and the black middle class of Tuskegee, Alabama, through the 1970s; see Manning Marable, "Tuskegee and the Politics of Illusion in the New South," *Black Scholar* 8 (May 1977): 13–24.

30. Ralph Ellison, *Invisible Man,* 2nd ed. (New York: Vintage International, 1995). Evidence of the actual Moton's classism can be found in reports of a pre-Study syphilis treatment program in Macon County, Georgia. Physicians from the PHS involved in that program were concerned that the high rate of syphilis—36 percent of all those tested—in Macon County might be embarrassing to the Institute. According to their reports of a meeting with him about their findings, Moton "calmly

stated he was surprised to find it did not run over 50 percent instead of 36"; Jones, *Bad Blood,* 76. Reverby discusses how the high rate of syphilis found by the PHS might have been the result of a localized outbreak in the southern part of the county; see Reverby, *Examining Tuskegee,* 35.

31. "Selected Letters between the United States Public Health Service, the Macon County Health Department, and the Tuskegee Institute, 1932–1972," in *Tuskegee's Truths,* ed. Susan M. Reverby (Chapel Hill: University of North Carolina Press, 2000). See also Reverby, *Examining Tuskegee,* 39–40.

32. Jones, *Bad Blood,* 100.

33. Jones, *Bad Blood,* 138.

34. Gray, *The Tuskegee Syphilis Study,* 74.

35. Jack Slater, "Condemned to Die for Science," *Ebony,* November 1972, 184. Susan Reverby claims that Ford used the Study as a campaign issue when he first ran for mayor; *Examining Tuskegee,* 132.

36. Slater, "Condemned to Die," 190.

37. Ellison, *Invisible Man,* 36.

38. Tuskegee Syphilis Study Legacy Committee. "Legacy Committee Request." In *Tuskegee's Truths: Rethinking the Tuskegee Syphilis Study,* edited by Susan M. Reverby (Chapel Hill, NC: University of North Carolina Pressm, 2000), 561. Reverby makes a similar claim, but she expands it to the town and to the civil rights legacy of the area; see *Examining Tuskegee,* 132.

39. William Jefferson Clinton, "Remarks by the President in Apology for the Study Done in Tuskegee," in Susan M. Reverby, *Tuskegee's Truths: Rethinking the Tuskegee Syphilis Study* (Chapel Hill: University of North Carolina Press, 2000), 575. Lynn Harter and colleagues also note that the remarks frame it as the "study *done in Tuskegee,*" which helps to redefine the roles of the town and the Institute; Harter, Stephens, and Japp, "President Clinton's Apology," 26.

Such naming conventions represent a challenge for scholarship on the Study. Outside of members of the Tuskegee University community and scholars delving into the history of the Study, alternate names are unfamiliar. One must refer to the "Tuskegee Syphilis Study" so readers *know* what is being discussed, and also because the name "Tuskegee Syphilis Study" reflects the memory narratives that have circulated since 1972. It also reflects, as will become apparent below, the naming conventions used by Fred Gray and the Tuskegee History Center in their discussion of the Study. As a result of these tensions, I have decided to use as much as possible the language of "the Study" or "the study done in Tuskegee" to capture the historical facts of the Study. I also use this language when discussing the Legacy Museum that makes use of similar nomenclature, but I also use "Tuskegee Syphilis Study" when discussing previous articulations of memory that used that name and when discussing the Tuskegee History Center that also uses that name for the Study.

40. Fred D. Gray, *Bus Ride to Justice* (Montgomery, AL: Black Belt Press, 1995).

41. For more on Sims and his research, see Margaret R. Brazier, "Exploitation and Enrichment: The Paradox of Medical Experimentation," *Journal of Medical Ethics* 34, no. 3 (2008); Robin E. Jensen, *Infertility: Tracing the History of a Transformative Term* (University Park, PA: Penn State University Press, 2016), 29–34.

42. Emphasis mine.

43. The lawyers are Charles Langford, Orzell Billingsley, Peter Hall, Arthur Shores, and Fred Gray.

44. The National Bar Association is an association of African American lawyers created in 1925, after several African American lawyers were denied entrance into the American Bar Association.

45. According to Manning Marable, African American electoral control of Macon County's local government led to "the subordination of municipal and county governments to the initiatives of the state government," a practice common across the South as African American politicians gained local political prominence; see Marable Manning, "Tuskegee and the Politics of Illusion in the New South," *Black Scholar* 8 (May 1977): 21.

46. The screens, in order of appearance, cover (1) the prehistory of Macon County (i.e., the time of the dinosaurs), (2) the removal of the Creek

Indians, (3) Booker T. Washington, (4) facts of the Tuskegee Syphilis Study, including audiovisual from *Dateline* and PBS features on Tuskegee from the early and mid-1990s, (5) a television playing C-SPAN footage of President Clinton's apology for the Study, (6) a screen about the National Bar Association (broken during the observation), (7) a screen that played a reenactment of the all-white group of lawyers and politicians who crafted Alabama's 1901 segregationist constitution, and (8) television coverage of protest marches and white backlash against them.

47. According to Susan Reverby, Gray was not invited to the initial meetings of the Syphilis Study Legacy Committee because it was funded by the CDC. Because Gray had sued the CDC and the federal government, he could not be invited to participate in a CDC-funded event; Reverby, *Examining Tuskegee,* 222.

48. Clinton, "Remarks by the President," 576.

49. According to a Tuskegee University website, the Bioethics Center was "officially established" in 1999 but did not open until 2006; see https://www.tuskegee.edu/about-us/centers-of-excellence/bioethics-center. The Legacy Museum opened in April 2009; see "The Legacy Museum," https://www.tuskegee.edu/libraries/legacy-museum.

50. "The Legacy Museum."

51. The content of the exhibits devoted to the Study and to HeLa cells remain largely the same. There is still a large amount of material in the first exhibit space devoted to George Washington Carver, but new material has been added, and additional key figures from the Institute's history are recognized in the new exhibit unveiled in 2017.

52. Since 2015 (the time of my initial visits to the Legacy Museum), some of the material devoted to Polk's photography has been replaced by other exhibits, which still feature Carver prominently.

53. An encounter with another staff member later in the day began with the declaration "The first thing you need to know is that it is *not* the 'Tuskegee Syphilis Study.' Tuskegee [Institute] had nothing to do with the Study. The government planned it. Only one of the autopsies was ever conducted here, and the rest were performed elsewhere!" According

to most accounts of the Study, the John A. Andrew Memorial Hospital was the site for the initial observations and medical tests performed on the men, including the one-time performance of lumbar punctures (aka "spinal taps"); see Gray, *The Tuskegee Syphilis Study*; Jones, *Bad Blood*; Reverby, *Examining Tuskegee*.

54. This claim, while novel, emphasizes the Institute's ignorance of the Study and has similarities to the 1972 press release by the Tuskegee Institute stating that the Institute's connection to the Study had been severed by the 1940s, when penicillin had become available for treating syphilis; see Jones, *Bad Blood*, 208.

55. In February 2015, the poster was not framed, as it was still being used at academic conferences. By December 2015, the poster was reprinted, framed, and hung in the gallery. A set of banners dividing the room and describing on one half the Tuskegee University Cooperative Extension Service were hung in the gallery.

56. The Legacy Museum, *The Patient, The Project, The Partnership* (Tuskegee, AL: Tuskegee University Library Services, 2012), 3. This pamphlet was part of the materials for the 2012 conference. I thank Jontyle Robinson, curator of the Legacy Museum, for providing me with a copy. For more on Henrietta Lacks and the HeLa cell line, see Rebecca Skloot, *The Immortal Life of Henrietta Lacks* (New York: Crown Publishers, 2010).

57. This was the only image of Henrietta Lacks in the exhibit in February 2015. During the First Bioethics Conference on Cancer Health Disparities Research, held January 18–20, 2012, this image was supplemented by a one-act play about Lacks. *Henrietta Lacks: Cellvation!* provided substantially more detail about Lacks's life, thus fleshing out the "patient" component of the exhibit's tripartite theme. I am thankful to Stephen Olufemi Sodeke, professor of allied health and bioethicist at the Tuskegee University National Center for Bioethics, for providing details about the conference and the one-act play. See also Stephen Olufemi Sodeke, "Introduction," *Journal of Health Care for the Poor and Underserved* 23, no. 4 (2014): 1–4.

58. In November 2015, the original poster describing the start of the partnership was replaced with framed posters describing some of the

scientific work done by the partnership, along with photographs of individuals involved in the partnership presenting at conferences, etc.

59. This is a key point in Paul Stob's recuperation of Washington; see Stob, "Black Hands Push Back," esp. 146–50.

60. Bernard J. Armada, "Memorial Agon: An Interpretive Tour of the National Civil Rights Museum," *Southern Communication Journal* 63, no. 3 (1998).

CHAPTER 4. MINIMAL REMEMBRANCE AND THE OBLIGATION
TO REMEMBER: OFFICIAL AND VERNACULAR MEMORIES
OF THE WILLOWBROOK STATE SCHOOL

1. *Willowbrook: The Last Great Disgrace,* http://index.geraldo.com/folio/willowbrook. The language of "profoundly and severely retarded" reflects the classifications of mental disability used in 1972, where profound and severe retardation were the two most severe categories of disability. When I am employing sources from previous decades, I will use the language that was in use at that time. Otherwise, I will use the language of "developmental disability" to describe those who resided at Willowbrook.

2. David J. Rothman and Sheila M. Rothman, *The Willowbrook Wars* (New York: Harper & Row, 1984), 45; James W. Trent Jr., *Inventing the Feeble Mind: A History of Mental Retardation in the United States* (Berkeley: University of California Press, 1994), 258.

3. "The Case of Willowbrook State Hospital Research: May 4, 1972," in *Symposium on Ethical Issues in Human Experimentation* (New York: Urban Health Affairs Program, New York University Medical Center, 1972), 4; Rothman and Rothman, *Willowbrook Wars,* 15–65.

4. The first eight years of the operation of the consent decree and the moving of residents into community housing settings is addressed in *Willowbrook Wars.* The remaining years are briefly addressed in David Goode et al., *A History and Sociology of the Willowbrook State School* (New York: American Association on Intellectual and Developmental Disabilities, 2013).

5. Henry K. Beecher, "Ethics and Clinical Research," *New England Journal of Medicine* 274, no. 24 (1966); "The Case of Willowbrook."

6. Jeffrey M. Cohen, "History and Ethics of Human Subjects Research," CITI Program, https://www.citiprogram.org; Bruce Gordon, "Vulnerable Subjects—Research Involving Children," CITI Program, https://www.citiprogram.org.

7. Carole Blair, Greg Dickinson, and Brian L. Ott, "Introduction: Rhetoric/Memory/Place," in *Places of Public Memory: The Rhetoric of Museums and Memorials,* ed. Greg Dickinson, Carole Blair, and Brian L. Ott (Tuscaloosa: University of Alabama Press, 2010), 7.

8. Trent, *Inventing the Feeble Mind;* Goode et al., *History and Sociology.*

9. Trent, *Inventing the Feeble Mind,* 250.

10. Trent, *Inventing the Feeble Mind,* 251.

11. For details on how institutions used their inmates or patients for labor, see Trent, *Inventing the Feeble Mind;* Goode et al., *History and Sociology.*

12. The percentages reported here come from Rothman and Rothman, *Willowbrook Wars,* 24.

13. Rothman and Rothman, *Willowbrook Wars,* 23.

14. Goode et al., *History and Sociology,* 71.

15. As Joel Howell and Rodney Hayward note, the highest infection rate identified in Krugman's studies in the 1950s was 25 infections in every 1,000 patients, aged 15–19 years, but Krugman and colleagues leapt from that rate to the belief that infection was "inevitable," a hunch that remained unproven until 1978; see Joel Howell and Rodney A. Hayward, "Writing Willowbrook, Reading Willowbrook: The Recounting of a Medical Experiment," in *Useful Bodies,* ed. Jordan Goodman, Anthony McElligott, and Lara Marks (Baltimore, MD: Johns Hopkins University Press, 2003).

16. The following description of the research conducted at Willowbrook is drawn from multiple sources, including "The Case of Willowbrook"; Daniel S. Gillmor, "How Much for the Patient? How Much for Medical Science? An Interview with Dr. Saul Krugman," *Modern Medicine* 30 (1974); Howell and Hayward, "Writing Willowbrook, Reading Willowbrook"; Saul Krugman, "The Willowbrook Hepatitis Studies

Revisited: Ethical Aspects," *Reviews of Infectious Diseases* 8, no. 1 (1986); Rothman and Rothman, *Willowbrook Wars;* Allen B. Weise, *Medical Odysseys: The Different and Sometimes Unexpected Pathways to Twentieth-Century Medical Discoveries* (New Brunswick, NJ: Rutgers University Press, 1991), 22–24.

17. At the time, there was no clear recognition of different viruses producing different types of hepatitis; it was viewed as the same disease expressed in slightly different forms.

18. Howell and Hayward note, somewhat ironically, the list of precautions the research team took to eliminate bacteria and other non-viral infectious agents from the mixture; Howell and Hayward, "Writing Willowbrook, Reading Willowbrook," 191.

19. Rothman, *Strangers at the Bedside,* 77; "1983 Award Winners," http://www. laskerfoundation.org/awards/1983_p_description.htm. A more extensive description of his more than twenty-five national and international awards can be found online at the NYU Health Sciences Library archive; see "Saul Krugman M.D.—Physician, Scientist, Teacher, 1911–1995," Lilian & Clarence de la Chapelle Medical Archives, https://archives.med. nyu.edu/exhibits/1292.

20. Weise, *Medical Odysseys,* 16. The other two men are Baruch Blumberg and Albert Prince.

21. Beecher, "Ethics and Clinical Research."

22. Materials from the protest actions by the Progressive Labor Party and the Medical Committee for Human Rights (MCHR) are part of the Willowbrook archival material held at the College of Staten Island; WSSM 7, box 1, folder 4. For more on the MCHR, see John Dittmer, *The Good Doctors: The Medical Committee for Human Rights and the Struggle for Social Justice in Health Care* (New York: Bloomsbury Press, 2009). For information on the Progressive Labor Party, see Max Elbaum, *Revolution in the Air* (New York: Verso, 2002), 63–72.

23. "The Case of Willowbrook."

24. See the presentation by Ellen Isaacs, "The Case of Willowbrook," 19–25.

25. Rothman and Rothman, *Willowbrook Wars,* 261. Similar points can be found in David J. Rothman, "Were Tuskegee and Willowbrook 'Studies in Nature'?," *Hastings Center Report* 12, no. 2 (1982).

26. Rothman and Rothman, *Willowbrook Wars,* 266.

27. Rothman and Rothman, *Willowbrook Wars,* 266–67.

28. "The Case of Willowbrook"; Gillmor, "How Much for the Patient?"; Krugman, "Willowbrook Hepatitis Studies Revisited."

29. Marita Sturken, *Tangled Memories* (Berkeley: University of California Press, 1997), 47.

30. For more on the qualities of monumental histories and memory, see Friedrich Nietzsche, *On the Advantage and Disadvantage of History for Life,* trans. Peter Preuss (Indianapolis, IN: Hackett Publishing, 1980), 17.

31. Jeffrey Olick argues that late nineteenth-century public memory, especially in Europe, deployed what I describe here as monumental forms; see Olick, *The Politics of Regret: On Collective Memory and Historical Responsibility* (New York: Routledge, 2007).

32. Building 2 had also housed Krugman's hepatitis research unit.

33. I heard the claim that Goode's publication spurred the creation of the path during a visit to CSI's campus in April 2015. For Goode et al.'s reference to the memorial, see Goode et al., *History and Sociology,* 299.

34. This practice still continues on the Office for Persons with Developmental Disabilities (OPWDD) campus that is located on the remainder of the old Willowbrook property.

35. Rothman and Rothman provide a well-detailed account of New York State's foot-dragging when it came to implementing this change; Rothman and Rothman, *Willowbrook Wars.*

36. The most notable exception is Bernard Carabello, a resident who suffered from cerebral palsy and who featured prominently in new coverage of Willowbrook in 1972.

37. Barbie Zelizer, "The Voice of the Visual in Memory," in *Framing Public Memory,* ed. Kendall Phillips (Tuscaloosa: University of Alabama Press, 2004), 162. See also Charles E. Scott, "The Appearance of Public Memory," in *Framing Public Memory,* ed. Kendall R. Phillips (Tuscaloosa: University of Alabama Press, 2004), 147–56.

38. The two-week-long display of the exhibit at the Museum of disABILITY History in Buffalo, New York, also included a crib that was standard for New York's large institutions for the developmentally disabled; see

"'Remembering Willowbrook' Exhibit Opening." http://youtu.be/vkmyPhY7Mw8.

39. Based on my visit to CSI and the former Willowbrook buildings, and a comparison of this image to those photographs I took during my visit, this last image is likely of Building 29's outdoor pavilion area. Three Willowbrook buildings—Buildings 25, 27, and 29, which according to architectural drawings of the school were to house "infirm males"—languish. Architectural drawings and maps are found at the CSI archive.

40. The photograph in its entirety is reprinted in Goode et al., *History and Sociology,* 98.

41. Beyond issues of budgets and systemic problems with OPWDD, there is the issue of trans-institutionalization, wherein individuals have been shifted from state hospitals to state prisons following the closure of state hospitals and facilities like Willowbrook; see Catherine Prendergast, "On the Rhetorics of Mental Disability," in *Embodied Rhetorics: Disability in Language and Culture,* ed. James C. Wilson and Cynthia Lewiecki-Wilson (Carbondale: Southern Illinois University Press, 2001), 52.

42. In addition to the stories about the school and the hepatitis experiments, Willowbrook is also recalled in connection with Andre Rand, who was convicted of kidnapping young children during the 1970s and 1980s and suspected in multiple missing-persons cases. Rand and Willowbrook also became linked to the urban legend of "Cropsey," a crazed killer roaming the New York City area. These linkages most likely occur because Rand had worked at Willowbrook in the 1960s and had made a makeshift campsite on the grounds of the school in the mid-80s.

43. Bill Nichols, *Introduction to Documentary* (Bloomington: Indiana University Press, 2001).

44. Michael J. Hyde, *The Life-Giving Gift of Acknowledgment* (West Lafayette, IN: Purdue University Press, 2006); see also Lisbeth Lipari, *Listening, Thinking, Being: Toward an Ethics of Attunement* (University Park, PA: Penn State University Press, 2014).

45. Neil Carter and John Williams, "'A Genuinely Emotional Week': Learning Disability, Sport and Television—Notes on the Special Olympics GB National Summer Games 2009," *Media, Culture & Society* 34,

no. 2 (2012): 218–20.

46. Jay Dolmage, *Disability Rhetoric,* Critical Perspectives on Disability (Syracuse, NY: Syracuse University Press, 2014), 42–43.

47. Rosemarie Garland Thomson, "Seeing the Disabled: Visual Rhetorics of Disability in Popular Photography," in *The New Disability History: American Perspectives,* ed. Paul K. Longmore and Lauri Umanski (New York: New York University Press, 2000), 341–42. See also Carter and Williams, "A Genuinely Emotional Week"; Dolmage, *Disability Rhetoric;* Keith Storey, "The Case against the Special Olympics," *Journal of Disability Policy Studies* 15, no. 1 (2004).

48. Goode et al., *History and Sociology;* Trent, *Inventing the Feeble Mind.*

49. Rothman and Rothman, *Willowbrook Wars,* 26–34; Trent, *Inventing the Feeble Mind,* 251–52.

50. Prendergast, "On the Rhetorics of Mental Disability."

51. Leslie Brenner, "Patti-Ann Gets a Beach House," *New York Magazine,* May 24, 1993, 18.

52. One of most organized and well-known groups of self-advocates are individuals on the autism spectrum; see the Autism Self-Advocacy Network, http://autisticadvocacy.org.

53. Sturken, *Tangled Memories,* 85. Television's "movie of the week" genre is also a popular vehicle for crafting public memory; see John A. Lynch, "Memory and Matthew Shepard: Opposing Expressions of Public Memory in Television Movies," *Journal of Communication Inquiry* 31, no. 3 (2007): 222–38.

54. It is notable that neither Dr. Horowitz nor Mrs. Sussman have their first names used in the film.

55. The choice of injection over ingestion might also reflect misunderstandings about how the research was conducted. Joel Howell and Rodney Hayward note that claims that hepatitis was injected are incorrect and that the misunderstanding allows defenders of Krugman to discount the critics by claiming they are ignorant about the study they protest. While this charge could be levied against Cohen's film, such claims would ignore the affective charge of depicting ingestion versus depicting injection. Second, it ignores the convoluted relationship

Krugman and his collaborators, especially Joan Giles, have with claims about their experiments. For example, Giles's letter to *The Lancet* attacking critics fosters the claim of injection: "For here is the truth: you cannot clinically tell the newly admitted child from the child injected"; Joan Giles, "Hepatitis Research among Retarded Children," *The Lancet* 279, no. 7709 (1971): 1126.

56. The use of "fantasia" here is distinct from the use of "fantasy" in some disability studies scholarship, where fantasy indicates a broad cultural formation driven by psychoanalytic impulses and anxieties. For examples of this use of "fantasy," see J. Preston, *The Fantasy of Disability: Images of Loss in Popular Culture* (Abingdon, UK: Taylor & Francis, 2016); Ellen Samuels, *Fantasies of Identification: Disability, Gender, Race* (New York: NYU Press, 2014).

57. Garland Thomson, "Seeing the Disabled," 341.

58. Garland Thomson, "Seeing the Disabled," 341.

59. For a description of the proposed Mile, see "The Willowbrook Mile Collaboration," http://csitoday.com/wp-content/uploads/2016/09/Willowbrook-Mile-Collaboration.pdf.

60. College of Staten Island, "Willowbrook Groundbreaking Ceremony," https://www.youtube.com/watch?v=3w7L9kScuLg.

CHAPTER 5. ATTEMPTING TO FORGET: THE UNIVERSITY OF CINCINNATI RADIATION STUDIES

1. This description of Saenger's radiation research and reactions to it in the introduction is drawn from multiple sources, including the Advisory Committee on Human Radiation Experiments (ACHRE), *Final Report* (Washington, DC: Advisory Committee on Human Radiation Experiments, 1995), 366–420; Gerald Kutcher, *Contested Medicine: Cancer Research and the Military,* large print ed. (Sydney, Australia: Read How You Want, 2010), 139–77; Eileen Welsome, *The Plutonium Files: America's Secret Medical Experiments in the Cold War* (New York: Dell Publishing, 1999), 337–51; Martha Stephens, *The Treatment: The Story of Those Who Died in the Cincinnati Radiation Tests* (Durham, NC: Duke University Press, 2002).

2. While these patients had cancer that would eventually be fatal, the research team reported to the DOD that the patients were in stable condition and that many were still working every day prior to radiation exposure.

3. Some details from these multiple reports eventually appeared in the ACHRE *Final Report* and can be found throughout Stephens's *The Treatment.* Copies of all the reports and many of the news stories on these events are found in the University of Cincinnati's Henry R. Winkler Center for the History of the Health Professions in the Whole Body Radiation Study and Eugene Saenger collections, respectively WBS and ES herein.

4. Carol Mason Spicer, "Fallout from Government-Sponsored Radiation Research," *Kennedy Institute of Ethics Journal* 4, no. 2 (1994).

5. In the original documentation, a range of names are used: Total Body Irradiation, Whole-Body Irradiation, and Whole Body Radiation, etc. The most consistent naming convention at the University of Cincinnati and in the archival materials is "Whole Body Radiation Study," which is used here.

6. Greg Dickinson, *Suburban Dreams: Imagining and Building the Good Life* (Tuscaloosa: University of Alabama Press, 2015), 128–30.

7. Stuart Auerbach and Thomas O'Toole, "Pentagon Has Contract to Test Radiation Effect on Humans," *Washington Post,* October 8, 1971.

8. Auerbach and O'Toole, "Pentagon Has Contract."

9. Eugene Saenger to Roger Rapoport, April 19, 1971, WBS 27. This letter in the WBS archival materials references an in-person conversation in October or November 1970, and an exchange of correspondence from November to April that was not found in the archive.

10. Roger Rapoport, *The Great American Bomb Machine* (New York: Ballantine Books, 1971).

11. Eugene Saenger to Arthur Newmyer, December 20, 1971, WBS 28. Arthur Newmyer was a lawyer in Washington, DC, who was hired by the University of Cincinnati to help manage fallout from the public disclosure of the study.

12. John Watson, "Defense Nuclear Agency Memo for Record," WBS 30;

Edward Silberstein and Eugene L. Saenger, "Ethics on Trial: Medical, Congressional, and Journalistic," unpublished essay, 1975, found in WBS 25.

13. "Kennedy to Investigate Radiation Test Project," *Washington Post,* October 9, 1971. See also Ellis Mottur interview, October 17, 2006, Edward M. Kennedy Oral History Project, Miller Center, University of Virginia, 17.

14. "Pentagon Pact for Study of Radiation Revealed," *Toledo Blade,* October 12, 1971.

15. Kutcher, *Contested Medicine;* Eugene Saenger, interview by Benjamin Felson and Charles Barrett, February 1984, Oral History of Medicine in Cincinnati, University of Cincinnati Library, Cincinnati, OH, https://ucl.mediaspace.kaltura.com/media/Eugene+Saenger+interviewed+by+Benjamin+Felson+and+Charles+Barrett%2C+February%2C+1984/1_bqzasrlt.

16. All quotations and paraphrases of the press conference are drawn from a transcript in the Whole Body Radiation Study files; WBS 27.

17. David J. Rothman, *Strangers at the Bedside* (New York: Basic Books, 1991), 168–84.

18. There are numerous inaccuracies, perhaps the most egregious being that the study had begun in 1955 prior to DOD funding, when in fact no element of the study began until a contract between the university and the DOD was secured and went into effect in 1960. This inaccurate statement appeared in subsequent news coverage and in the testimony John Northrop of the Defense Nuclear Agency prepared for a Senate Subcommittee on Health hearing that was never held; see draft statement by John Northrop, November 1971, WBS 27; "Pentagon Pact for Study of Radiation Revealed"; "Pentagon's Radiation Study Defended," *Washington Post,* October 12, 1971. Further details on the various inaccuracies in the press release can be found in Kutcher, *Contested Medicine,* 274–81.

19. Edward Gall to Joyce Endejann, October 25, 1971, ES 12:271. Similar sentiments can be found in a memo summarizing a phone call between Charles Barrett and Senator Robert Taft's Senate office, October 12, 1971, box 171, folder 5, Robert Taft, Jr. Papers, Manuscript Division, Library of Congress, Washington, DC (hereafter "Taft Papers").

20. Edward Silberstein and Eugene L. Saenger, "Ethics on Trial: Medical, Congressional, and Journalistic" (1975), 7; WBS 25.

21. A copy of this letter is found in correspondence between Saenger and Robert McConnell and Otha Linton of the ACR; WBS 25. Kutcher reports that Gravel contacted the ACR after his request for an inquiry into the Cincinnati study was rebuffed by the surgeon general and the American Cancer Society; Kutcher, *Contested Medicine,* 282n39.

22. Otha Linton to Sen. Mike Gravel, blind carbon copy to Eugene Saenger, November 24, 1971, WBS 27.

23. Robert McConnell to Sen. Mike Gravel, January 4, 1972, page 1, WBS 28.

24. Robert McConnell to Sen. Mike Gravel, January 4, 1972, page 2, WBS 28.

25. Robert McConnell to Sen. Mike Gravel, January 4, 1972, page 3, WBS 28.

26. Lew Moores, "Radiation Project Stopped until Committee Reports," *UC News Record,* February 1, 1972. A *New York Times* article in 1994 revealed that at the time of the ACR investigation, Saenger sat "on five of the organization's subcommittees and commissions. Dr. Robert W. McConnell, the group's president, was a fishing buddy and signed the investigative report." See Keith Schneider, "Cold War Radiation Test on Humans to Undergo a Congressional Review," *New York Times,* April 11, 1994.

27. Bennis emphasizes this in a February 16 letter to Senator Kennedy, which was also copied to Sen. Robert Taft, Jr.; see Warren Bennis to Edward Kennedy, February 16, 1972, box 171, folder 6, Taft Papers. See also Dan Aylward, "Blue-Ribbon Committee Recommends Changes," *UC News-Record,* February 1, 1972; Moores, "Radiation Project Stopped."

28. Moores, "Radiation Project Stopped"; Stephens, *The Treatment,* 92–98.

29. Moores, "Radiation Project Stopped."

30. Aylward, "Blue-Ribbon Committee"; "Continue Radiation Project, UC Advised," *Cincinnati Post,* February 2, 1972.

31. Memo from Raymond Suskind to members of the Ad Hoc Committee-Radiation Study, February 12, 1972, ES 2:143.

32. Memo from Raymond Suskind to members of the Ad Hoc Committee-Radiation Study, February 12, 1972, ES 2:143.

33. The *UC News Record,* the student-run newspaper at the University of Cincinnati, published several articles in February about the conflicts of interest on the committee, including Dr. Aron's role in the WBS study; see Moores, "Radiation Project Stopped"; Lew Moores, "Suskind Comm.—Conflict of Interest," *UC News Record,* February 11, 1972.

34. Edward Gall to Warren Bennis, January 26, 1972, ES 12:84; Raymond Suskind to Warren Bennis, February 7, 1972, ES 1:6–8; Ed Gall to unknown, April 11, 1972, WBS 32; Bennis to Gall, April 24, 1972, WBS 32; Vernon Stroud to Robert O'Neil, April 24, 1972, WBS 32; Robert O'Neil to Vernon Stroud, April 24, 1972, WBS 32.

35. Junior Faculty Association (JFA), *A Report to the Campus Community* (hereafter "JFA report"), 1, WBS 28. A copy of the JFA report is also in the papers of Robert Taft Jr.; see Taft Papers, box 171, folder 6.

36. JFA report, 1–2, WBS 28.

37. William Bozman, "UC Faculty Group Would End Whole Body Radiation Program," *Cincinnati Enquirer,* January 26, 1972; Tommy West, "UC Would Limit Radiation Patients," *Cincinnati Enquirer,* February 3, 1972.

38. "Kennedy to Investigate Radiation Test Project." See also Ellis Mottur Interview, October 17, 2006, Edward M. Kennedy Oral History Project, Miller Center, University of Virginia, 17.

39. Rothman, *Strangers at the Bedside,* 168–88.

40. Pat Gwaltney to Sen. Robert Taft, Jr., November 2, 1971, box 171, folder 5, Taft Papers. John Northrop of the Defense Nuclear Agency (which funded Saenger's research) also prepared testimony to present to Kennedy's Health Subcommittee, but there is no indication it was delivered; see draft testimony of John Northrop, WBS 27, and Eugene Saenger to John Northrop, November 26, 1971, WBS 27.

41. Memorandum by Edward Silberstein, December 6, 1971, WBS 27.

42. Memorandum by Eugene Saenger, December 6, 1971, WBS 27; Kutcher discusses how Saenger here viewed the request to interview patients as an affront to his professional respectability and authority as a physician; see

Kutcher, *Contested Medicine,* 295–96.

43. Susan Reverby indicates that the testimony of the survivors of the Tuskegee Syphilis Study—and a vocal African American constituency protesting it—were necessary components to the finally successful legislative push to regulate research; see Reverby, *Examining Tuskegee: The Infamous Syphilis Study and Its Legacy,* reprint (Chapel Hill: University of North Carolina Press, 2009), 101–103, 191.

44. Edward Silberstein to Edward Gall, December 9, 1971, WBS 27; emphasis mine.

45. Eugene Saenger to Charles Barrett, December 17, 1971, WBS 32. See also Eugene Saenger to Edward Gall, December 11, 1971, WBS 27; and Eugene Saenger to Edward Gall, December 21, 1971, WBS 28.

46. Edward Gall to Senator Edward Kennedy, December 22, 1971, box 176, folder 5, Taft Papers.

47. University of Cincinnati General Counsel to Warren Bennis, January 4, 1972, WBS 32.

48. University of Cincinnati General Counsel to Warren Bennis, January 4, 1972, WBS 32.

49. Robert Webb, "Kennedy Aide Says UC Refusal Endangers Funds for Research," *Cincinnati Enquirer,* January 4, 1972.

50. Sen. Edward Kennedy to Warren Bennis, January 11, 1971, WBS 28. See also Robert Webb, "UC Admits NET Filmed 3 Radiation Patients," *Cincinnati Enquirer,* January 15, 1972; "UC Restudying Position on Probe by Senate," *Cincinnati Post,* January 15, 1972.

51. Webb, "UC Admits NET Filmed"; Eugene Saenger to Edward Gall, January 13, 1972, WBS 28. Prior to the *Washington Post* story on October 8, Saenger was quite willing to facilitate interviews of patients with interested journalists; see, e.g., Eugene Saenger to Roger Rapoport, April 19, 1971, WBS 27.

52. Eugene Saenger to Edward Gall, January 13, 1972, WBS 28.

53. Eugene Saenger to Edward Gall and Charles Barrett, January 14, 1972, WBS 28.

54. "UC Restudying Position"; "Kennedy May Yet Get Look at UC Project," *Cincinnati Enquirer,* January 25, 1972.

55. Edward Gall to Sen. Edward Kennedy, January 19, 1972, WBS 28.

56. Joseph Ross to Edward Gall, February 10, 1972, WBS 28; B. J. Kennedy to Edward Gall, February 14, 1972, WBS 28.

57. U.S. Congress, *Congressional Record,* 92nd Congress, 2nd sess., 1972, S. 12373–76; James Grohl, "Human Experiment Controls Included in Senate Bill," *Cincinnati Post,* August 2, 1972; James Grohl, "Pentagon Didn't Fund UC Program, Report Given Kennedy in May Shows," *Cincinnati Post,* August 2, 1972.

58. Stephens, *The Treatment,* 12.

59. Randal F. Kleine, "Gilligan Joins in Radiation Controversy," *UC News Record,* March 7, 1972.

60. Yet Martha Stephens did have access to retrospective accounts from 1994 by John Gilligan that indicated no plans were made to shutter the study at this meeting. Her collections of news clippings from the 1990s are in box 2, folder 1, Martha Stephens Papers, University of Cincinnati Libraries. Gilligan's recollection is reported in two articles in the *Cincinnati Enquirer:* Paul Barton and Howard Wilkinson, "Ex-Aide: Taft Blocked UC Probe," *Cincinnati Enquirer,* February 9, 1994; Howard Wilkinson, "UC 'Stiff-Armed' Investigators," *Cincinnati Enquirer,* February 9, 1994.

61. Kennedy to Gilligan, February 24, 1972, box 171, folder 6, Taft Papers.

62. Notes by Robert Taft, February 25, 1972, box 171, folder 6, Taft Papers.

63. Wilkinson, "UC 'Stiff-Armed' Investigators."

64. Silberstein to undisclosed recipients, January 18, 1972, WBS 28.

65. See discussion in chapter 2.

66. Silberstein also conducted interviews with three of the participants or their family members about possible contact with Kennedy's office. These interviews are conducted in front of other members of the research team and the radiation department who were involved in the interviewee's cancer treatment. Silberstein asks them if *he and the research team members who are present* have treated them like human guinea pigs. In the face of such a coercive setting, it should be unsurprising that all the participants said they were not treated like guinea pigs and would not like to be interviewed. He also informed the participants that "they had a constitutional right to say anything they wished about us or nothing."

Interview transcripts by Edward Silberstein, WBS 28; Silberstein to Gall, January 12, 1972, WBS 28. For a similar view of this issue, see Kutcher, *Contested Medicine,* 301–2.

67. Edward Gall to Ellis Mottur, January 25, 1972, box 171, folder 6, Taft Papers.

68. Saenger, Charles Barrett, and other UC officials also reached out to others in Ohio's congressional delegation, including Cincinnati-area Congressman Charles Keating and Senator William Saxbe (through the intermediary of department-store magnate Simon Lazarus Jr.). Keating and Saxbe were also Republicans. See Eugene Saenger to Mike Gertner [Saxbe aide], January 29, 1972, WBS 28; Edward Kennedy to Charles Keating, January 20, 1972, box 171, folder 6, Taft Papers; Clifford Grulee to Edward Gall, January 28, 1972 [a memo about contact with Rep. Keating's office], ES 10:144.

69. In notes for a first-person narrative he was writing in the mid-'90s, Saenger indicates that there was "much contact between ELS [Saenger] and Taft" and that his cousin Jack Martin was a staffer for Taft; ES box 1, folder 5. In a 2006 oral history interview, Ellis Mottur says that Saenger "happened to be the doctor who treated all of Senator Bob Taft, Jr.'s relatives for cancer, so Senator Taft had a very close personal relationship with that doctor and just loved him." Ellis Mottur interview, October 17, 2006, Edward M. Kennedy Oral History Project, Miller Center, University of Virginia, 19. I have not been able to verify the specifics of Mottur's claims, but they help reinforce that a close connection of some sort existed between Taft and Saenger.

70. Ellis Mottur interview, October 17, 2006, Edward M. Kennedy Oral History Project, Miller Center, University of Virginia, 19.

71. Memo by unknown for Robert Taft, October 12, 1971, box 171, folder 5, Taft Papers. The memo also notes the university's desire to keep the story "'low key' unless absolutely forced to do otherwise."

72. Rady Johnson (DOD) to Robert Taft, Jr., October 14, 1971, box 171, folder 5, Taft Papers; Robert Taft, Jr. to Rady Johnson, October 18, 1971, box 171, folder 5, Taft Papers; Pat Gwaltney to Robert Taft, Jr., November 2, 1971, box 171, folder 5, Taft Papers; Edward Kennedy to

Robert Taft, Jr., December 11, 1971, box 171, folder 5, Taft Papers; Robert Taft, Jr., to Edward Kennedy, December 11, 1971, box 171, folder 5, Taft Papers; Notes by Robert Taft, December 14, 1971, box 171, folder 5, Taft Papers.

73. Memo by unknown, December 15, 1971, box 171, folder 5, Taft Papers.

74. Floor speech by Robert Taft, Jr., presentation copy with annotations, box 171, folder 5, Taft Papers.

75. Floor speech by Robert Taft, Jr., presentation copy with annotations; box 171, folder 5, Taft Papers.

76. "Taft Attacks Cincy U. Rap by Kennedy," *Cleveland Plain-Dealer,* December 16, 1971; "Taft Asks UC Hearings," *Akron News,* December 16, 1971; "Taft Asks Hearing on Cancer Unit," *Toledo Blade,* December 16, 1971; "Taft Rakes Ted's UC Inquiry," *Dayton Journal-Herald,* December 16, 1971; Robert Webb, "Taft Rips Kennedy's UC Probe," *Cincinnati Enquirer,* December 16, 1971; "Taft Asks Subcommittee Hearings on Cincinnati Cancer Treatment," *Columbus Dispatch,* December 16, 1971; "Taft Raps Kennedy's Cincy Probe," *Columbus Citizen-Journal,* December 16, 1971.

77. Memo by unknown, undated, box 171, folder 5, Taft Papers. While there is no direct indication of which statement Barrett is referencing on the memo, the memo itself is included with a series of handwritten notes by Taft and a partial draft of the December 15th statement with handwritten comments and additions on it. Given the tenor of the speech he delivered, it seems plausible that Barrett was talking about this statement.

78. Robert Webb, "Senate's Cancer Probe Widens," *Cincinnati Enquirer,* December 17, 1971. Taft's call for hearings was also mentioned by Kennedy during his meeting with Governor Gilligan, Bennis, and Barrett on February 24; see notes by Robert Taft, February 25, 1972, box 171, folder 6, Taft Papers.

79. Taft to Kennedy, December 23, 1971, box 171, folder 5, Taft Papers.

80. Memo by Bill Wickens, December 23, 1971, WBS 28; Undated memo by unknown, box 171, folder 5, Taft Papers.

81. Taft to Kennedy, January 4, 1972, box 171, folder 6, Taft Papers. A copy can also be found in the UC WBS archive, WBS 28.

82. Scott Allen, "Kennedy Dropped Testing Probe; Taft's Anger Led to 1971 Decision," *Boston Globe,* February 12, 1994, quoted in Robert Martin, "Interviewer's Briefing Materials for Ellis Mottur Interview," in Edward M. Kennedy Oral History Project, Miller Center, University of Virginia, 2006.

83. Kennedy to Senate Health Subcommittee, July 25, 1972, box 171, folder 6, Taft Papers.

84. Undated memo, box 171, folder 6, Taft Papers. Although undated, the references to the amendment and the DOD not being concerned about the amendment in the memo strongly indicate that this conversation was in reference to the July 25 request for co-sponsorship and occurred sometime in late July or early August of 1972.

85. Bradford Gray to Raymond Suskind, October 16, 1972, ES 7:199.

86. Suskind to Gray, October 22, 1974, ES 7:198.

87. Gray to Suskind, October 30, 1974, ES 7:197.

88. Gray to Suskind, October 30, 1974, ES 7:197.

89. Suskind to Gray, November 4, 1974, ES 7:195–96.

90. Gray to Suskind, November 8, 1974, box 1, folder 36, Martha Stephens Papers.

91. Suskind to Gray, November 15, 1974, box 1, folder 36, Martha Stephens Papers.

92. Silberstein and Saenger, "Ethics on Trial."

93. Stephens, *The Treatment,* 103–4.

94. Silberstein and Saenger to Otha Linton, Robert McConnell, Warren Bennis, Edward Gall, and Charles Bennett, May 8, 1975, WBS 25. Form letters to other recipients of the essay manuscript can be found in the Whole Body Study archive with identical language.

95. William Beierwaltes to Eugene Saenger, May 19, 1975, WBS 25. Martha Stephens notes that Beierwaltes misunderstood the purposes of the research, believing it focused on leukemia, which was treated with whole body radiation, instead of radioresistant tumors, which were not treated with whole body radiation; see Stephens, *The Treatment,* 103. A similar confusion about the research can be found in the response of B. J. Kennedy; see B. J. Kennedy to Silberstein, May 16, 1975, WBS 25.

96. Charles Barrett to Silberstein and Saenger, May 15, 1975, WBS 25; Robert McConnell to Silberstein and Saenger, May 20, 1975, WBS 25.

97. Saenger to Warren Bennis, July 5, 1975, WBS 25.

98. Beierwaltes to Saenger, May 19, 1975, WBS 25.

99. Gall to Silberstein, January 28, 1975, WBS 25.

100. Otha Linton to Silberstein, May 27, 1975, WBS 25.

101. U.S. Congress, House Committee on Energy and Commerce, Subcommittee on Energy Conservation and Power, *American Nuclear Guinea Pigs: Three Decades of Radiation Experiments on U.S. Citizens,* 99th Congress, 2nd sess. Reports on the minimal—and misleading—journalistic accounts of the report can be found in Geoffrey Sea, "The Radiation Story No One Would Touch," *Columbia Journalism Review* 32, no. 6 (1994). In recounting previous studies of radiation experiments, the ACHRE *Final Report* (xxii) describes *American Nuclear Guinea Pigs* as "virtually forgotten."

102. Spicer, "Fallout."

103. Nick Miller, "The Secret History of UC's Radiation Tests," *Cincinnati Post,* January 29, 1994.

104. A copy of Executive Order 12891 creating the ACHRE is found in the final report; Advisory Committee on Human Radiation Experiments (ACHRE), *Final Report,* 859–61.

105. ACHRE, *Final Report,* chapter 4.

106. Paul Barton, "Saenger's Tests May Be Probed More Closely," *Cincinnati Enquirer,* September 20, 1994.

107. Paul Barton, "Tilt in Favor of Saenger Charged," *Cincinnati Enquirer,* August 2, 1994; see also Stephens, *The Treatment,* 123.

108. ACHRE, *Final Report,* 405.

109. ACHRE, *Final Report,* 773.

110. ACHRE, *Final Report,* 804.

111. Marcus Paroske, "Deliberating International Science Policy Controversies: Uncertainty and AIDS in South Africa," *Quarterly Journal of Speech* 95 (2009): 151. See also Leah Ceccarelli, "Manufactured Scientific Controversy: Science, Rhetoric, and Public Debate," *Rhetoric & Public Affairs* 14, no. 2 (2011).

112. Allen Buchanan, "The Controversy over Retrospective Moral Judgment,"

Kennedy Institute of Ethics Journal 6, no. 3 (1996): 245–50. Several other members or staff of ACHRE discussed the disagreements that constituted an epistemological filibuster, although they do not use that language. See Tom L. Beauchamp, "Looking Back and Judging Our Predecessors," *Kennedy Institute of Ethics Journal* 6, no. 3 (1996): 251–70; Ruth Macklin, "Disagreement, Consensus, and Moral Integrity," *Kennedy Institute of Ethics Journal* 6, no. 3 (1996): 289–311; R. Alta Charo, "Commentary: Principles and Pragmatism," *Kennedy Institute of Ethics Journal* 6, no. 3 (1996): 319–22.

113. Complaint, In re Cincinnati Radiation, 874 F. Supp. 796 (S.D. Ohio 1995) (No. 1:94-cv-00126). In re Cincinnati Radiation, Docket No. 1:94-cv-00126 (S.D. Ohio, Feb. 17, 1994).

114. Stephens, *The Treatment,* 232. See also Linda Dono Reeves, "Radiation Suit Claims Denial of Civil Rights," *Cincinnati Enquirer,* February 18, 1994. For a list of all plaintiffs and defendants, see In re Cincinnati Radiation.

115. Additional details about the lawsuit can be found in Stephens, *The Treatment,* chapters 11–13.

116. Paul Barton, "Radiation Lawsuit Settled," *Cincinnati Enquirer,* August 29, 1996.

117. Charles E. Morris III, "My Old Kentucky Homo: Lincoln and the Politics of Queer Public Memory," in *Framing Public Memory,* ed. Kendall R. Phillips (Tuscaloosa: University of Alabama Press, 2004), 99n34.

118. Memorandum and Order, In re Cincinnati Radiation, 2 (C-1-94-126), August 4, 1997, box 1, folder 2, ES collection; see also Barton, "Radiation Lawsuit Settled."

119. Description of memorial plaque, box 3, folder 13, Martha Stephens Papers.

120. Memorandum and Order, In re Cincinnati Radiation, 2 (C-1-94-126), August 4, 1997, box 1, folder 2, ES collection.

121. Memorandum and Order, In re Cincinnati Radiation, 5 (C-1-94-126), October 27, 1997, box 1, folder 2, ES collection; see also Stephens, *The Treatment,* 283. Only 70 of the 88 names were included as some families "did not want their relative's names included"; see Marie McCain, "Plaque Doesn't End Pain of UC Radiation Case," *Cincinnati Enquirer,*

October 9, 1999.

122. Tim Bonfield, "Radiation Controversy Outlasts Lawsuit," *Cincinnati Enquirer,* October 9, 1999.

123. Bonfield, "Radiation Controversy."

124. McCain, "Plaque Doesn't End Pain."

125. Tim Bonfield, "Part of Hospital Demolished; Pavilion J Housed Cancer Experiment," *Cincinnati Enquirer,* June 11, 2001.

126. Bonfield, "Part of Hospital Demolished."

127. Jeff Jacobson, personal communication, August 8, 2016.

128. Carl Elliot, "How the University of Cincinnati Buries Its Sins," *Fear and Loathing in Bioethics* (blog), June 14, 2017, http://loathingbioethics. blogspot.com/2017/06/how-university-of-cincinnati-buries-its.html.

129. Lisa Smith, "Out-of-the-Way Memorial Remembers Cincinnati Patients Who Died in Radiation Testing," broadcast, *WCPO News* (Cincinnati, OH: WCPO, July 3, 2017).

130. Smith, "Out-of-the-Way Memorial."

131. Smith, "Out-of-the-Way Memorial."

Conclusion

1. Arthur W. Frank, "Truth Telling, Companionship and Witness: An Agenda for Narrative Bioethics," *Hastings Center Report* 46, no. 3 (2016): 18.

2. Carole Blair, Greg Dickinson, and Brian L. Ott, "Introduction: Rhetoric/Memory/Place," in *Places of Public Memory: The Rhetoric of Museums and Memorials,* ed. Greg Dickinson, Carole Blair, and Brian L. Ott (Tuscaloosa: University of Alabama Press, 2010), 16.

3. Thomas G. Benedek and Jonathon Erlen, "The Scientific Environment of the Tuskegee Study of Syphilis, 1920–1960," *Perspectives in Biology and Medicine* 43, no. 1 (1999); Robert M. White, "Unraveling the Tuskegee Syphilis Study," *Arthritis Care & Research* 47, no. 4 (2002).

4. James Jones argues that the physicians at the U.S. Public Health Service did *not* defend the study, unlike Saul Krugman at Willowbrook and Saenger at Cincinnati, because they recognized the racist implications of their work; see James H. Jones, *Bad Blood: The Tuskegee Syphilis Experiment*

(New York: Free Press, 1993), 201–2.

5. John A. Lynch, "Memory and Matthew Shepard: Opposing Expressions of Public Memory in Television Movies," *Journal of Communication Inquiry* 31, no. 3 (2007).

6. Kendall R. Phillips, "The Failure of Memory: Reflections on Rhetoric and Public Remembrance," *Western Journal of Communication* 74, no. 2 (2010): 219.

7. Sarah J. L. Edwards, "Assessing the Remedy: The Case for Contracts in Clinical Trials," *American Journal of Bioethics* 11, no. 4 (2011).

8. David Rothman discusses the ways paternalism persists in the epilogue to *Strangers at the Bedside* (New York: Basic Books, 1991), 247–62.

9. Eric Juengst et al., "From 'Personalized' to 'Precision' Medicine: The Ethical and Social Implications of Rhetorical Reform in Genomic Medicine," *Hastings Center Report* 46, no. 5 (2016): 22.

10. Juengst et al., "From 'Personalized' to 'Precision' Medicine," 27.

11. Tom L. Beauchamp and James Childress, *Principles of Biomedical Ethics,* 7th ed. (New York: Oxford University Press, 2013).

12. Marion Danis, Yolanda Wilson, and Amina White, "Bioethicists Can and Should Contribute to Addressing Racism," *American Journal of Bioethics* 16, no. 4 (2016). See also Kayhan Parsi, "The Unbearable Whiteness of Bioethics," *American Journal of Bioethics* 16, no. 4 (2016).

13. See Beauchamp and Childress, *Principles of Biomedical Ethics; Belmont Report,* available at http://www.hhs.gov/ohrp/regulations-and-policy/belmont-report/index.html#xbasic.

14. Rebecca Skloot, *The Immortal Life of Henrietta Lacks* (New York: Crown Publishers, 2010); Margaret R. Brazier, "Exploitation and Enrichment: The Paradox of Medical Experimentation," *Journal of Medical Ethics* 34, no. 3 (2008).

15. Brazier, "Exploitation and Enrichment"; Soloman R. Benatar, "Justice and Medical Research: A Global Perspective," *Bioethics* 15, no. 4 (2001); Merle Spriggs, "Canaries in the Mines: Children, Risk, Non-Therapeutic Research, and Justice," *Journal of Medical Ethics* 30 (2004).

16. For more on the Kennedy Krieger study, see Spriggs, "Canaries in the Mines."

References

———•◆•———

Advisory Committee on Human Radiation Experiments (ACHRE). *Final Report*. Washington, DC: Advisory Committee on Human Radiation Experiments, 1995.

Ahmed, Sara. *The Cultural Politics of Emotion*. New York: Routledge, 2004.

Akron News. "Taft Asks UC Hearings." December 16, 1971.

Allen, Scott. "Kennedy Dropped Testing Probe; Taft's Anger Led to 1971 Decision." *Boston Globe,* February 12, 1994.

Anderson, Warren D. "Outside Looking In: Observations on Medical Education since the Flexner Report." *Medical Education* 45 (2011): 29–35.

Armada, Bernard J. "Memorial Agon: An Interpretive Tour of the National Civil Rights Museum." *Southern Communication Journal* 63, no. 3 (1998): 235–43.

Arras, John D. "The Jewish Chronic Disease Hospital Case." In *The Oxford Textbook of Clinical Research Ethics,* edited by Ezekiel Emmanuel, Christine C. Grady, Robert A. Crouch, Reidar K. Lie, Franklin G. Miller, and David

D. Wendler, 73–79. New York: Oxford University Press, 2011.

Auerbach, Stuart, and Thomas O'Toole. "Pentagon Has Contract to Test Radiation Effect on Humans." *Washington Post,* October 8, 1971.

Aylward, Dan. "Blue-Ribbon Committee Recommends Changes." *UC News-Record,* February 1, 1972, 1.

Barr, Donald A. "Revolution or Evolution? Putting the Flexner Report in Context." *Medical Education* 45 (2011): 17–22.

Barton, Paul. "Radiation Lawsuit Settled." *Cincinnati Enquirer,* August 29, 1996.

——. "Saenger's Tests May Be Probed More Closely." *Cincinnati Enquirer,* September 20, 1994.

——. "Tilt in Favor of Saenger Charged." *Cincinnati Enquirer,* August 2, 1994.

Barton, Paul, and Howard Wilkinson. "Ex-Aide: Taft Blocked UC Probe." *Cincinnati Enquirer,* February 9, 1994.

Beauchamp, Tom L. "Looking Back and Judging Our Predecessors." *Kennedy Institute of Ethics Journal* 6, no. 3 (1996): 251–70.

Beauchamp, Tom L., and James Childress. *Principles of Biomedical Ethics.* 7th ed. New York: Oxford University Press, 2013.

Beecher, Henry K. "Ethics and Clinical Research." *New England Journal of Medicine* 274, no. 24 (1966): 1354–60.

Benatar, Soloman R. "Justice and Medical Research: A Global Perspective." *Bioethics* 15, no. 4 (2001): 333–40.

Benedek, Thomas G., and Jonathon Erlen. "The Scientific Environment of the Tuskegee Study of Syphilis, 1920–1960." *Perspectives in Biology and Medicine* 43, no. 1 (1999): 1–30.

Blair, Carole, Greg Dickinson, and Brian L. Ott. "Introduction: Rhetoric/Memory/Place." In *Places of Public Memory: The Rhetoric of Museums and Memorials,* edited by Greg Dickinson, Carole Blair, and Brian L. Ott, 1–54. Tuscaloosa: University of Alabama Press, 2010.

Bodnar, John. *Remaking America: Public Memory, Commemoration, and Patriotism in the Twentieth Century.* Princeton, NJ: Princeton University Press, 1992.

Bonfield, Tim. "Part of Hospital Demolished; Pavilion J Housed Cancer Experiment." *Cincinnati Enquirer,* June 11, 2001.

——. "Radiation Controversy Outlasts Lawsuit." *Cincinnati Enquirer,* October 9, 1999.

Bozman, William. "UC Faculty Group Would End Whole Body Radiation Program." *Cincinnati Enquirer,* January 26, 1972.

Brandt, Allen M. "Racism and Research: The Case of the Tuskegee Syphilis Experiment." In *Tuskegee's Truths: Rethinking the Tuskegee Syphilis Study,* edited by Susan M. Reverby, 15–33. Chapel Hill: University of North Carolina Press, 2000.

Brandt, Allen M., and Lara Freidenfelds. "Research Ethics after World War II: The Insular Culture of Biomedicine." *Kennedy Institute of Ethics Journal* 6, no. 3 (1996): 239–43.

Brazier, Margaret R. "Exploitation and Enrichment: The Paradox of Medical Experimentation." *Journal of Medical Ethics* 34, no. 3 (2008): 180–83.

Brody, Howard, and Mark Clark. "Narrative Ethics: A Narrative." *Hastings Center Report* 44, no. 1 (2014): S7–S11.

Browne, Stephen. "Reading Public Memory in Daniel Webster's *Plymouth Rock Oration.*" *Western Journal of Communication* 57 (1993): 464–77.

———. "Reading, Rhetoric and Texture of Public Memory." *Quarterly Journal of Speech* 81 (1995): 237–51.

Buchanan, Allen. "The Controversy over Retrospective Moral Judgment." *Kennedy Institute of Ethics Journal* 6, no. 3 (1996): 245–50.

Carter, Neil, and John Williams. "'A Genuinely Emotional Week': Learning Disability, Sport and Television—Notes on the Special Olympics GB National Summer Games 2009." *Media, Culture & Society* 34, no. 2 (2012): 211–27.

"The Case of Willowbrook State Hospital Research: May 4, 1972." In *Symposium on Ethical Issues in Human Experimentation.* New York: Urban Health Affairs Program, New York University Medical Center, 1972.

Casey, Edward S. "Public Memory in Place and Time." In *Framing Public Memory,* edited by Kendall R. Phillips, 17–44. Tuscaloosa: University of Alabama Press, 2004.

Ceccarelli, Leah. "Manufactured Scientific Controversy: Science, Rhetoric, and Public Debate." *Rhetoric & Public Affairs* 14, no. 2 (2011): 195–228.

———. *On the Frontier of Science: An American Rhetoric of Exploration and Exploitation.* East Lansing: Michigan State University Press, 2013.

Charo, R. Alta. "Commentary: Principles and Pragmatism." *Kennedy Institute of*

Ethics Journal 6, no. 3 (1996): 319–22.

Cincinnati Enquirer. "Kennedy May Yet Get Look at UC Project." January 25, 1972.

Cincinnati Post. "Continue Radiation Project, UC Advised." February 2, 1972.

———. "UC Restudying Position on Probe by Senate." January 15, 1972.

Cleveland Plain-Dealer. "Taft Attacks Cincy U. Rap by Kennedy." December 16, 1971.

Cochrane, Rexmond C. *The National Academy of Sciences: The First Hundred Years, 1863-1963.* Washington, DC: National Academies Press, 1978.

Cohen, Jeffrey M. "History and Ethics of Human Subjects Research." CITI Program, https://www.citiprogram.org.

Columbus Citizen-Journal. "Taft Raps Kennedy's Cincy Probe." December 16, 1971.

Columbus Dispatch. "Taft Asks Subcommittee Hearings on Cincinnati Cancer Treatment." December 16, 1971.

Cvetkovich, Ann. *Depression: A Public Feeling.* Durham, NC: Duke University Press, 2012.

Danis, Marion, Yolanda Wilson, and Amina White. "Bioethicists Can and Should Contribute to Addressing Racism." *American Journal of Bioethics* 16, no. 4 (2016): 3–12.

Dayton Journal-Herald. "Taft Rakes Ted's UC Inquiry." December 16, 1971.

Dickinson, Greg. *Suburban Dreams: Imagining and Building the Good Life.* Tuscaloosa: University of Alabama Press, 2015.

Dickinson, Greg, Brian L. Ott, and Eric Aoki. "Memory and Myth at the Buffalo Bill Museum." *Western Journal of Communication* 69, no. 2 (2005): 85–108.

———. "Spaces of Remembering and Forgetting: The Reverent Eye/I at the Plains Indian Museum." *Communication and Critical/Cultural Studies* 3, no. 1 (2006): 27–47.

Dittmer, John. *The Good Doctors: The Medical Committee for Human Rights and the Struggle for Social Justice in Health Care.* New York: Bloomsbury Press, 2009.

Dolmage, Jay. *Disability Rhetoric.* Critical Perspectives on Disability. Syracuse, NY: Syracuse University Press, 2014.

Dresser, Rebecca. "Personal Knowledge and Study Participation." *Journal of Medical Ethics* 40 (2014): 471–74.

Dubriwny, Tasha, and Kristan Poirot, eds. "Gender and Public Memory." Special issue. *Southern Communication Journal* 82, no. 4 (2017): 3–12.

Dunn, Thomas R. "Remembering 'a Great Fag': Visualizing Public Memory and the Construction of Queer Space." *Quarterly Journal of Speech* 97, no. 4 (2011): 435–60.

———. "Remembering Matthew Shepard: Violence, Identity and Queer Counterpublic Memories." *Rhetoric & Public Affairs* 13, no. 4 (2010): 611–52.

Eberly, Rosa. "'Everywhere You Go, It's There': Forgetting and Remembering the University of Texas Tower Shooting." In *Framing Public Memory,* edited by Kendall R. Phillips, 65–88. Tuscaloosa: University of Alabama Press, 2004.

Edwards, Sarah J. L. "Assessing the Remedy: The Case for Contracts in Clinical Trials." *American Journal of Bioethics* 11, no. 4 (2011).

Elbaum, Max. *Revolution in the Air.* New York: Verso, 2002.

Elliot, Carl. "How the University of Cincinnati Buries Its Sins." In *Fear and Loathing in Bioethics.* Blog. June 14, 2017. http://loathingbioethics.blogspot.com.

Ellison, Ralph. *Invisible Man.* 2nd ed. New York: Vintage International, 1995.

Faden, Ruth, and Tom L. Beauchamp. *A History and Theory of Informed Consent.* New York: Oxford University Press, 1986.

Fletcher, John C. "Clinical Bioethics at the NIH: History and a New Vision." *Kennedy Institute of Ethics Journal* 5, no. 4 (1995): 355–64.

Frank, Arthur W. "Truth Telling, Companionship and Witness: An Agenda for Narrative Bioethics." *Hastings Center Report* 46, no. 3 (2016): 17–21.

Freidenfelds, Lara. "Recruiting Allies for Reform: Henry Knowles Beecher's 'Ethics and Clinical Research.'" *International Anesthesiology Clinics* 45, no. 4 (2007): 79–103.

Gallagher, Victoria J. "Memory and Reconciliation in the Birmingham Civil Rights Institute." *Rhetoric & Public Affairs* 2, no. 2 (1999): 303–20.

Garland Thomson, Rosemarie. "Seeing the Disabled: Visual Rhetorics of Disability in Popular Photography." In *The New Disability History: American Perspectives,* edited by Paul K. Longmore and Lauri Umanski, 335–74. New York: NYU Press, 2000.

Garver, Eugene. *Aristotle's Rhetoric: An Art of Character.* Chicago: University of

Chicago Press, 1994.

Giles, Joan. "Hepatitis Research among Retarded Children." *The Lancet* 279, no. 7709 (1971): 1126.

Gillmor, Daniel S. "How Much for the Patient? How Much for Medical Science? An Interview with Dr. Saul Krugman." *Modern Medicine* 30 (1974): 30–35.

Goode, David, Darryl Hill, Jean Reiss, and William Bronston. *A History and Sociology of the Willowbrook State School.* New York: American Association on Intellectual and Developmental Disabilities, 2013.

Goodman, Jordan, Anthony McElligott, and Lara Marks. "Making Human Bodies Useful: Historicizing Medical Experiments in the Twentieth Century." In *Useful Bodies,* edited by Jordan Goodman, Anthony McElligott, and Lara Marks, 1–23. Baltimore, MD: Johns Hopkins University Press, 2003.

Gray, Fred D. *Bus Ride to Justice.* Montgomery, AL: Black Belt Press, 1995.

——. *The Tuskegee Syphilis Study: The Real Story and Beyond.* Montgomery, AL: NewSouth Books, 1998.

Grohl, James. "Human Experiment Controls Included in Senate Bill." *Cincinnati Post,* August 2, 1972.

——. "Pentagon Didn't Fund UC Program, Report Given Kennedy in May Shows." *Cincinnati Post,* August 2, 1972.

Halpern, Jodi. "What Is Clinical Empathy?" *Journal of General Internal Medicine* 18, no. 8 (2003): 670–74.

Harris, Sheldon H. *Factories of Death: Japanese Biological Warfare, 1932–45, and the American Cover-up.* New York: Routledge, 1994.

Harter, Lynn M., Ronald J. Stephens, and Phyllis M. Japp. "President Clinton's Apology for the Tuskegee Syphilis Experiment: A Narrative of Remembrance, Redefinition, and Reconciliation." *Howard Journal of Communications* 11 (2000): 19–34.

Hasian, Marouf, Jr. "Remembering and Forgetting the 'Final Solution': A Rhetorical Pilgrimage to the Holocaust Museum." *Critical Studies in Media Communication* 21, no. 1 (2004): 64–92.

Hasian, Marouf. "Authenticity, Public Memories, and the Problematics of Post-Holocaust Remembrances: A Rhetorical Analysis of the

Wilkomirski Affair." *Quarterly Journal of Speech* 91, no. 3 (2005): 231–63.

Hawhee, Debra. "Rhetoric's Sensorium." *Quarterly Journal of Speech* 101, no. 1 (2015): 2–17.

Heidegger, Martin. *Being and Time.* Translated by John Macquarrie and Edward Robinson. New York: Harper & Row, 1962.

Heller, Jean. "Syphilis Victims in U.S. Study Went Untreated for 40 Years." In *Tuskegee's Truths: Rethinking the Tuskegee Syphilis Study,* edited by Susan M. Reverby, 116–18. Chapel Hill: University of North Carolina Press, 2000.

Herzig, Rebecca M. *Suffering for Science: Reason and Sacrifice in Modern America.* New Brunswick, NJ: Rutgers University Press, 2005.

Hoerl, Kristen. "Burning Mississippi into Memory: Cinematic Amnesia as a Resource for Civil Rights." *Critical Studies in Media Communication* 26, no. 1 (2009): 54–79.

Howell, Joel, and Rodney A. Hayward. "Writing Willowbrook, Reading Willowbrook: The Recounting of a Medical Experiment." In *Useful Bodies,* edited by Jordan Goodman, Anthony McElligott, and Lara Marks, 190–213. Baltimore, MD: Johns Hopkins University Press, 2003.

Hyde, Michael J. *The Call of Conscience: Heidegger and Levinas, Rhetoric and the Euthanasia Debate.* Columbia: University of South Carolina Press, 2001.

———. *The Life-Giving Gift of Acknowledgment.* West Lafayette, IN: Purdue University Press, 2006.

Jensen, Robin E. *Infertility: Tracing the History of a Transformative Term.* University Park, PA: Penn State University Press, 2016.

Johnson, Jenell. "'A Man's Mouth Is His Castle': The Midcentury Fluoridation Controversy and the Visceral Public." *Quarterly Journal of Speech* 102, no. 1 (2016): 1–20.

Jones, David S., Christine C. Grady, and Susan E. Lederer. "'Ethics and Clinical Research'—the 50th Anniversary of Beecher's Bombshell." *New England Journal of Medicine* 374 (2016): 2393–98.

Jones, James H. *Bad Blood: The Tuskegee Syphilis Experiment.* New York: Free Press, 1993.

———. "Foreword." In *Tuskegee's Truths: Rethinking the Tuskegee Syphilis Study,* edited by Susan M. Reverby, xiii-xxi. Chapel Hill: University of North Carolina Press, 2000.

Juengst, Eric, Michelle L. McGowan, Jennifer R. Fishman, and Richard A. Settersen Jr. "From 'Personalized' to 'Precision' Medicine: The Ethical and Social Implications of Rhetorical Reform in Genomic Medicine." *Hastings Center Report* 46, no. 5 (2016): 21–33.

Kadushin, Charles. "Social Distance between Client and Professional." *American Journal of Sociology* 67, no. 5 (1962): 517–31.

Kang, Lydia, and Nate Pedersen. *Quackery: A Brief History of the Worst Ways to Cure Everything.* New York: Workman Publishing Co., 2017.

Katriel, Tamar. "Sites of Memory: Discourses of the Past in Israeli Pioneering Settlement Museums." *Quarterly Journal of Speech* 80, no. 1 (1994): 1–20.

Keränen, Lisa. "The Hippocratic Oath as Epideictic Rhetoric: Reanimating Medicine's Past for Its Future." *Journal of Medical Humanities* 22, no. 1 (2001): 55–68.

Klein, Kerwin Lee. "On the Emergence of Memory in Historical Discourse." *Representations* 69 (2000): 127–50.

Kleine, Randal F. "Gilligan Joins in Radiation Controversy." *UC News Record,* March 7, 1972.

Krugman, Saul. "The Willowbrook Hepatitis Studies Revisited: Ethical Aspects." *Reviews of Infectious Diseases* 8, no. 1 (1986): 157–62.

Kuhn, Thomas. *The Structure of Scientific Revolutions.* 2nd ed. Chicago: University of Chicago Press, 1970.

Kutcher, Gerald. *Contested Medicine: Cancer Research and the Military.* Large print ed. Sydney, Australia: Read How You Want, 2010.

Lederer, Susan. *Subjected to Science: Human Experimentation in America before the Second World War.* Baltimore, MD: Johns Hopkins University Press, 1995.

Leontsini, Eleni. "The Motive of Society: Aristotle on Civic Friendship, Justice, and Concord." *Res Publica* 19, no. 1 (2013): 21–35.

Lindberg, David C. *The Beginnings of Western Science: The European Scientific Tradition in Philosophical, Religious, and Institutional Context, 600 B.C. to A.D. 1450.* Chicago: University of Chicago Press, 1992.

Lipari, Lisbeth. *Listening, Thinking, Being: Toward an Ethics of Attunement.* University Park, PA: Penn State University Press, 2014.

Ludmerer, Kenneth M. "Abraham Flexner and Medical Education." *Perspectives in Biology and Medicine* 54, no. 1 (2011): 8–16.

Lynch, John A. "Memory and Matthew Shepard: Opposing Expressions of Public Memory in Television Movies." *Journal of Communication Inquiry* 31, no. 3 (2007): 222–38.

Lynch, John A., and Mary E. Stuckey. "'This Was His Georgia': Polio, Poverty, and Public Memory at FDR's Little White House." *Howard Journal of Communications* 28, no. 4 (2017): 390–404.

Macklin, Ruth. "Disagreement, Consensus, and Moral Integrity." *Kennedy Institute of Ethics Journal* 6, no. 3 (1996): 289–311.

Marable, Manning. "Tuskegee and the Politics of Illusion in the New South." *Black Scholar* 8 (May 1977): 13–24.

Massumi, Brian. *Parables for the Virtual: Movement, Affect, Sensation.* Durham, NC: Duke University Press, 2002.

McCain, Marie. "Plaque Doesn't End Pain of UC Radiation Case." *Cincinnati Enquirer,* October 9, 1999.

McCarthy, Charles R. "The Origins and Policies That Govern Institutional Review Boards." In *The Oxford Textbook of Clinical Research Ethics,* edited by Ezekiel Emmanuel, Christine C. Grady, Robert A. Crouch, Reidar K. Lie, Franklin G. Miller, and David D. Wendler, 541–51. New York: Oxford University Press, 2011.

Miller, Lynn E., and Richard M. Weiss. "Revisiting Black Medical School Extinctions in the Flexner Era." *Journal of the History of Medicine and Allied Sciences* 67, no. 2 (2011): 217–43.

Miller, Nick. "The Secret History of UC's Radiation Tests." *Cincinnati Post,* January 29, 1994.

Montello, Martha. "Narrative Ethics." *Hastings Center Report* 44, no. 1 (2014): S2–S6.

Moores, Lew. "Radiation Project Stopped until Committee Reports." *UC News Record,* February 1, 1972.

———. "Suskind Comm.—Conflict of Interest." *UC News Record,* February 11, 1972.

Morris, Charles E., III. "My Old Kentucky Homo: Lincoln and the Politics of Queer Public Memory." In *Framing Public Memory,* edited by Kendall R. Phillips, 89–114. Tuscaloosa: University of Alabama Press, 2004.

———, ed. *Remembering the AIDS Quilt.* East Lansing: Michigan State University

Press, 2011.

———. "Sunder the Children: Abraham Lincoln's Queer Rhetorical Pedagogy." *Quarterly Journal of Speech* 99, no. 4 (2013): 395–422.

Nichols, Bill. *Introduction to Documentary.* Bloomington: Indiana University Press, 2001.

Nietzsche, Friedrich. *On the Advantage and Disadvantage of History for Life.* Translated by Peter Preuss. Indianapolis, IN: Hackett Publishing, 1980.

Olansky, Sidney, Lloyd Simpson, and Stanley H. Schuman. "Environmental Factors in the Tuskegee Study of Untreated Syphilis." *Public Health Reports* 69, no. 7 (1954): 691–98.

Olick, Jeffrey K. "Collective Memory: The Two Cultures." *Sociological Theory* 17, no. 3 (1999): 333–48.

———. *The Politics of Regret: On Collective Memory and Historical Responsibility.* New York: Routledge, 2007.

Ott, Brian L., Eric Aoki, and Greg Dickinson. "Ways of (Not) Seeing Guns: Presence and Absence at the Cody Firearms Museum." *Communication & Critical/Cultural Studies* 8, no. 3 (2011): 215–39.

Page, Douglas, and Adrian Baranchuk. "The Flexner Report: 100 Years Later." *International Journal of Medical Education* 1 (2010): 74–75.

Paroske, Marcus. "Deliberating International Science Policy Controversies: Uncertainty and AIDS in South Africa." *Quarterly Journal of Speech* 95 (2009): 148–70.

Parsi, Kayhan. "The Unbearable Whiteness of Bioethics." *American Journal of Bioethics* 16, no. 4 (2016): 1–2.

Phillips, Kendall R. "The Failure of Memory: Reflections on Rhetoric and Public Remembrance." *Western Journal of Communication* 74, no. 2 (2010): 208–23.

———. "Introduction." In *Framing Public Memory,* edited by Kendall R. Phillips, 1–14. Tuscaloosa: University of Alabama Press, 2004.

Poirot, Kristan, and Shevaun E. Watson. "Memories of Freedom and White Resilience: Place, Tourism, and Urban Slavery." *Rhetoric Society Quarterly* 45, no. 2 (2015): 91–116.

Prendergast, Catherine. "On the Rhetorics of Mental Disability." In *Embodied Rhetorics: Disability in Language and Culture,* edited by James C. Wilson and Cynthia Lewiecki-Wilson, 45–60. Carbondale: Southern Illinois University Press, 2001.

Preston, J. *The Fantasy of Disability: Images of Loss in Popular Culture*. Abingdon, UK: Taylor & Francis, 2016.

Rapoport, Roger. *The Great American Bomb Machine*. New York: Ballantine Books, 1971.

Reeves, Linda Dono. "Radiation Suit Claims Denial of Civil Rights." *Cincinnati Enquirer,* February 18, 1994.

Reverby, Susan M. *Examining Tuskegee: The Infamous Syphilis Study and Its Legacy*. Reprint. Chapel Hill: University of North Carolina Press, 2009.

——. "Invoking 'Tuskegee': Problems in Health Disparities, Genetic Assumptions, and History." *Journal of Health Care for the Poor and Underserved* 21 (2010): 26–40.

——. "Listening to Narratives from the Tuskegee Syphilis Study." *The Lancet* 377 (2011): 1646–47.

——. "More Than Fact and Fiction: Cultural Memory and the Tuskegee Syphilis Study." *Hastings Center Report* 31, no. 5 (2001): 22–28.

——, ed. *Tuskegee's Truths*. Chapel Hill: University of North Carolina Press, 2000.

Reyes, G. Mitchell, ed. *Public Memory, Race, and Ethnicity*. Newcastle upon Tyne, UK: Cambridge Scholars Publishing, 2010.

Ridings, James E. "The Thalidomide Disaster: Lessons from the Past." In *Teratogenicity Testing*, vol. 947, *Methods in Molecular Biology (Methods and Protocols)*, edited by Paul C. Barrow, 575–86. Totowa, NJ: Humana Press, 2013.

Rothman, David J. *Strangers at the Bedside*. New York: Basic Books, 1991.

——. "Were Tuskegee and Willowbrook 'Studies in Nature'?" *Hastings Center Report* 12, no. 2 (1982): 5–7.

Rothman, David J., and Sheila M. Rothman. *The Willowbrook Wars*. New York: Harper & Row, 1984.

Samuels, Ellen. *Fantasies of Identification: Disability, Gender, Race*. New York: NYU Press, 2014.

Schneider, Keith. "Cold War Radiation Test on Humans to Undergo a Congressional Review." *New York Times,* April 11, 1994.

Schwartz, Barry, and Howard Schuman. "History, Commemoration, and Belief: Abraham Lincoln in American Memory, 1945–2001." *American Sociological Review* 70 (2005): 183–203.

Scott, Charles E. "The Appearance of Public Memory." In *Framing Public Memory*, edited by Kendall R. Phillips, 147–56. Tuscaloosa: University of Alabama Press, 2004.

Sea, Geoffrey. "The Radiation Story No One Would Touch." *Columbia Journalism Review* 32, no. 6 (1994): 37–40.

Skloot, Rebecca. *The Immortal Life of Henrietta Lacks*. New York: Crown Publishers, 2010.

Slater, Jack. "Condemned to Die for Science." *Ebony*, November 1972, 177–90.

Smith, Lisa. "Out-of-the-Way Memorial Remembers Cincinnati Patients Who Died in Radiation Testing." *WCPO News*. Broadcast. Cincinnati, OH: WCPO, July 3, 2017.

Sodeke, Stephen Olufemi. "Introduction." *Journal of Health Care for the Poor and Underserved* 23, no. 4 (2014): 1–4.

Spicer, Carol Mason. "Fallout from Government-Sponsored Radiation Research." *Kennedy Institute of Ethics Journal* 4, no. 2 (1994): 147–54.

Spriggs, Merle. "Canaries in the Mines: Children, Risk, Non-Therapeutic Research, and Justice." *Journal of Medical Ethics* 30 (2004): 176–81.

Stahnisch, Frank W., and Marja Verhoef. "The Flexner Report of 1910 and Its Impact on Complementary and Alternative Medicine and Psychiatry in North America in the 20th Century." *Evidence-Based Complementary and Alternative Medicine* 2012, Article ID 647896 (2012): 1–10.

Stephens, Martha. *The Treatment: The Story of Those Who Died in the Cincinnati Radiation Tests*. Durham, NC: Duke University Press, 2002.

Stob, Paul. "Black Hands Push Back: Reconsidering the Rhetoric of Booker T. Washington." *Quarterly Journal of Speech* 104, no. 2 (2018): 145–65.

Storey, Keith. "The Case against the Special Olympics." *Journal of Disability Policy Studies* 15, no. 1 (2004): 35–42.

Stormer, Nathan. *Sign of Pathology: U.S. Medical Rhetoric on Abortion, 1800s–1960s*. University Park, PA: Penn State University Press, 2015.

Sturken, Marita. *Tangled Memories*. Berkeley: University of California Press, 1997.

Thelan, David. "Memory and American History." *Journal of American History* 75

(1989): 1117–29.

Thomas, Stephen B., and Sandra Crouse Quinn. "Light on the Shadow of the Syphilis Study at Tuskegee." *Health Promotion & Practice* 1, no. 3 (2000): 234–37.

Thomas, Stephen B., and Sandra Crouse Quinn. "The Tuskegee Syphilis Study, 1932–1972: Implications for HIV Education and Aids Risk Education Programs in the Black Community." In *Tuskegee's Truths: Rethinking the Tuskegee Syphilis Study,* edited by Susan M. Reverby, 404–17. Chapel Hill, NC: University of North Carolina Press, 2000.

Toledo Blade. "Pentagon Pact for Study of Radiation Revealed." October 12, 1971.

——. "Taft Asks Hearing on Cancer Unit." December 16, 1971.

Trent, James W., Jr. *Inventing the Feeble Mind: A History of Mental Retardation in the United States.* Berkeley: University of California Press, 1994.

Tseng, Wei-Ting, and Ya-Ping Lin. "'Detached Concern' of Medical Students in a Cadaver Dissection Course: A Phenomenological Study." *Anatomical Sciences Education* 9, no. 3 (2015): 265–71.

Tuskegee Syphilis Study Legacy Committee. "Legacy Committee Request." In *Tuskegee's Truths: Rethinking the Tuskegee Syphilis Study,* edited by Susan M. Reverby, 559–66. Chapel Hill, NC: University of North Carolina Press, 2000.

Vivian, Bradford J. *Commonplace Witnessing: Rhetorical Invention, Historical Remembrance, and Public Culture.* New York: Oxford University Press, 2017.

——. "Jefferson's Other." *Quarterly Journal of Speech* 88 (2002): 284–302.

——. *Public Forgetting: The Rhetoric and Politics of Beginning Again.* State College, PA: Penn State University Press, 2010.

Washington, Booker T. "Cotton States Exposition Address." In *American Rhetorical Discourse,* edited by Ronald F. Reid, 565–67. Prospect Heights, IL: Waveland Press, 1995.

Washington Post. "Kennedy to Investigate Radiation Test Project." October 9, 1971.

——. "Pentagon's Radiation Study Defended." October 12, 1971.

Webb, Robert. "Kennedy Aide Says UC Refusal Endangers Funds for Research." *Cincinnati Enquirer,* January 4, 1972.

———. "Senate's Cancer Probe Widens." *Cincinnati Enquirer,* December 17, 1971.

———. "Taft Rips Kennedy's UC Probe." *Cincinnati Enquirer,* December 16, 1971.

———. "UC Admits NET Filmed 3 Radiation Patients." *Cincinnati Enquirer,* January 15, 1972.

Weise, Allen B. *Medical Odysseys: The Different and Sometimes Unexpected Pathways to Twentieth-Century Medical Discoveries.* New Brunswick, NJ: Rutgers University Press, 1991.

Welsome, Eileen. *The Plutonium Files: America's Secret Medical Experiments in the Cold War.* New York: Dell Publishing, 1999.

West, Tommy. "UC Would Limit Radiation Patients." *Cincinnati Enquirer,* February 3, 1972.

White, Robert M. "Unraveling the Tuskegee Syphilis Study." *Arthritis Care & Research* 47, no. 4 (2002): 457–58.

Wilkinson, Howard. "UC 'Stiff-Armed' Investigators." *Cincinnati Enquirer,* February 9, 1994.

Williams, Robert R. "Aristotle and Hegel on Recognition and Friendship." In *The Plural States of Recognition,* edited by Michel Seymour, 20–36. New York: Palgrave Macmillan, 2010.

Wilson, Kirt H. "Debating the Great Emancipator: Abraham Lincoln and Our Public Memory." *Rhetoric & Public Affairs* 13, no. 3 (2010): 455–80.

Wright, Elizabethada A. "Rhetorical Spaces in Memorial Places: The Cemetery as a Rhetorical Space/Place." *Rhetoric Society Quarterly* 25, no. 4 (2005): 51–81.

Young, James Harvey. *The Medical Messiahs: A Social History of Health Quackery in the Twentieth Century.* Expanded paperback ed. Princeton, NJ: Princeton University Press, 1992.

Zelizer, Barbie. "Reading the Past against the Grain: The Shape of Memory Studies." *Critical Studies in Mass Communication* 12 (1995): 214–39.

———. *Remembering to Forget: Holocaust Memory through the Camera's Lens.* Chicago: University of Chicago Press, 1998.

———. "The Voice of the Visual in Memory." In *Framing Public Memory,* edited by Kendall R. Phillips, 157–86. Tuscaloosa: University of Alabama Press, 2004.

Index